W9-CFH-423

ADVANCE REVIEWS

"People are very good at forgetting, which is why a book like this is so important. In *Open Heart Runner*, Gregory Marchand reminds us of many things: our fragility, our capacity for love, our deep desire for meaning. He reminds us that we are neither wholly flesh nor wholly spirit, but a strange amalgam of the two. *Open Heart Runner* rends the thin veil between our quotidian lives and a realm that connects us all, and teaches us *to love that well, which [we] must leave ere long.*"
　　—Terence Young, Governor-General's-Award-nominated
　　　poet and author of the novel *After Goodlake's*

"Gregory Marchand takes us to a place most of us will never be, or would chose to go. He re-enters life with rich insights that can help us all on our journey down the right road."
　　—Rob Reid, Race Director of the Royal Victoria Marathon

"Gregory Marchand's memoir centers on two equal and opposite lessons. The first is that of an endurance athlete, a longtime long-distance runner in his case, isn't guaranteed perfect cardiac health. Medical catastrophes can visit even the very fit. Greg's other lesson is that the human body and mind, with assists from advanced medical science, have amazing powers to rebound, even from life-threatening crises. Marchand's story is at first frightening and ultimately uplifting."
　　—Joe Henderson, author, running coach and
　　　former chief editor of *Runner's World* magazine

Open
Heart
Runner

searching for
meaning after
my heart stopped

Gregory Marchand

For Alex,
    With gratitude and heart-felt
Warmth.
                    Greg

Agio
PUBLISHING HOUSE

PUBLISHING HOUSE

151 Howe Street, Victoria BC Canada V8V 4K5

© 2012, Gregory Marchand.
All rights reserved.
Without limiting the rights under copyright reserved above,
no part of this publication may be reproduced, stored
in or introduced into a retrieval system, or transmitted,
in any form or by any means (electronic, mechanical,
photocopying, recording or otherwise), without the prior
written permission of both the copyright owner and the
publisher of this book.

For rights information and bulk orders, please contact
info@agiopublishing.com
or go to
www.agiopublishing.com

Visit Gregory Marchand's website at
www.openheartrunner.com

Open Heart Runner
ISBN 978-1-897435-79-3 (trade paperback)
ISBN 978-1-897435-78-6 (ebook)

Cataloguing information available from
Library and Archives Canada.
Printed on acid-free paper.
Agio Publishing House is a socially responsible company,
measuring success on a triple-bottom-line basis.
10 9 8 7 6 5 4 3 2 1c

For my parents, Pat and Lou;
my sisters, Luanne, Colette and Allison;
my wife, Debbie;
and my children, Lucas, Raechel and Leo.

And for all those who run and walk through life
with an open heart.

PROLOGUE

TERRORS

Something's wrong. I can feel it. I can't tell what it is, though. I've felt like this before. Or something like it. I always hurt when I run a race. Especially at the end. It's cold today and I just need to finish. But it hurts. I'm not breathing right.

Just get past it. That's all I need to do. This little climb to the finish line is nothing. I can even pass that woman just ahead of me. That would be good. Just a few more steps.

There's something wrong, though. My chest. My heart. I can't feel my arms. My fingers are tingling in my gloves. I feel tired. I am tired.

It hurts. I hurt.

I'm on the ground. What's going on? My head aches. My face hurts. I must have hit my head on something, on the gravel maybe. If I could just get up, I'd be okay.

I can't move. All these people around me. What's going on? I'm just tired. Let me get up. Let me move.

If you'd let me move, I'd be okay. The race is over. I'm okay.

When I was younger, starting at about eight or nine, I'd frequently wake my parents in the middle of the night crying out from a dream I was having. They'd hear me running around the house screaming. I was still asleep, or at least I was unconscious. But I was running, running away from something. My parents would chase after me trying to keep me from hurting myself and trying to calm me down enough to bring me back to reality.

Later, I wouldn't remember any of this. I wouldn't remember running, or screaming, or my parents chasing me. I'd only become aware of them and myself once they'd managed to slow me down, stop me from running, and give me a drink of water, the coolness of the liquid easing me back to reality as it ran down my throat.

Gradually, I'd wake up, my heart racing and sweat pouring down my face. I'd still be breathing hard, trying to understand what was going on and what I was feeling.

After I'd awakened fully, I'd start to remember the feeling that had pervaded my dream and started these night terrors. In my dream, I'd be aware of a darkness closing in on me. It was formless but large, like a pulsating blob of ink expanding around me. It would contract slightly then expand again even larger.

As I breathed, it would grow and surround me almost entirely. The more I breathed, the more it grew and the more I felt entrapped. I couldn't get away from it, so I'd run. But the harder I ran and the harder I breathed, the larger it grew. I didn't realize that if I just stopped running, I would breathe slower and allow the blob to fully contract and disappear.

But I was afraid. I wanted to escape it, not understanding that my only escape was to relax, to let go, to let it pass.

That same inkiness enveloped me as I lay on the ground at the end of the race surrounded by strangers pumping on my chest, breathing into my mouth, trying to push life into my lifeless body. As in my dream, I wanted to get up and run. Their hands pounding on my chest and their lips pressing against my mouth were too close. But my breath wouldn't come and the same blob of pressure that would surround me in my dreams entrapped me now, pushing on my chest, holding me down. I needed to get up. I needed to run away.

1

RACING

"Oh, be quiet," I muttered.

The buzz of the alarm clock pierced my sleep. I reached over to the table at my bedside, turned off the alarm, and lay back on my pillow not wanting to open my eyes.

My wife, Debbie, stirred beside me. "What time is it?" Her voice sounded groggy and slightly perturbed.

"Eight o'clock."

"Why so early? It's Sunday."

"The run."

"Oh, right."

Finally, I opened my eyes. Our bedroom was still dark, the sun, like Debbie and me, not yet risen. I pulled the quilt covering our bed back over my shoulders. It was so cold in the room that my fingers began to feel numb from the few seconds my arm had been uncovered.

"It's too cold," Debbie said.

"I know. The forecast is for snow later today."

"You're not really going to run, are you?"

"Well, I don't feel much like getting out of bed."

"Then don't."

"I've already registered for the race. I might as well run it."

"I'm going back to sleep."

I had no idea what lay ahead for me as I reluctantly climbed out of bed that morning. We all intellectually understand that our lives can change in an instant – that losing control of the car on a snow-covered road, eating poorly cooked food, or walking across thin ice on a frozen river can have consequences that are completely unexpected. I used to imagine what it would be like if my life suddenly altered course completely beyond my control. Now I know.

The chill shocked me as my feet touched the fir flooring of our bedroom. January can be cold in most parts of Canada, but Victoria is different. It's not supposed to be cold here, even in the winter. But the temperature had dropped below freezing overnight, and our 85-year-old home was not coping well with the cold as the morning dawned clear but brisk. Although I'd grown up on the stark Alberta prairie where winters can be deadly, I'd become accustomed to the temperate climate of Victoria. A chilly, January morning run held little attraction for me.

At least that's how I probably felt. I have only vague memories of January 11th, 1998. My conscious knowledge of the day has come from the reports of family and friends.

My son, Lucas, was 15 at the time, and we had planned to run the race together that morning. He and I had been running together since he was eight years old. At first I would run an easy pace to allow him to keep up. Now, he had become nothing more than the back of a flapping jersey as he consistently outran me. For the past week, he had been nursing a case of strep throat with antibiotics. I had registered him to run in the race anyway hoping he would be better by the weekend. But when I went downstairs to his room that morning to check on him and heard his laboured breathing, I knew he was still too sick to run. Today, I'm grateful he wasn't at the end of the race to see me collapse, to see my heart stop, to see my life fade.

Do all runners feel a need to run?

According to Debbie, I considered not running that morning as well. I'd recently cut my teaching load to part time, was supplementing my income working as a freelance writer, and had completed a busy week meeting several deadlines for writing assignments. It would have been nice to relax into a Sunday morning of reading the newspaper and sipping coffee without having to drive 20 kilometres to Saanichton and then run in the below-freezing temperature for eight kilometres. But then a friend called wondering if I planned to run the race. Later, he confided that he had hoped I would talk him out of running. But we were both driven by the undeclared notion that the other truly wanted to run. We agreed to meet at the fairgrounds.

I loved running. But, like anyone who participates in an activity that takes effort, I would often have to convince myself to actually do it. I looked forward to the exhilaration of the endorphin rush from running, but I often had to remind myself of that feeling in order to get myself started. Especially on a cold, January morning.

The race started at 11:00 a.m. After a light breakfast, I set out at about 10:00. I'd run the same race in past years so the route was familiar to me. The Saanichton Fairgrounds, where the race begins and ends, is a 20-minute drive from our home. The grounds are used for several community events, most notably the Labour Day weekend fair that attracts several thousand visitors viewing everything from home preserves and prized piglets to handmade quilts and oil paintings. In January, it's little more than a parking lot. That evening, long after the race had been completed, my brother-in-law was dispatched to pick up my car. It was in the middle of that darkened parking lot, a solitary vehicle looking abandoned by its driver.

I must have parked in the midst of several hundred other cars that morning and entered the main building to pick up my race packet. Inside, I talked to some other runners. A friend later interviewed many of those people.

One of those he interviewed, Merrell Harlow, was handing out registration packets and greeted me inside. Merrell was an avid runner, even in her fifties, and a long-time friend who worked at the school where I still teach.

"Where's Lucas?" she asked as I picked up my race packet.

When I told her that Lucas was sick, I admitted that I wasn't feeling great myself.

"Can anyone feel well in this weather?" she asked.

I must have finally braved the cold, leaving the warmth of the hall to join the more than 600 other runners outside. There I met a fellow writer and teacher, Marilyn McCrimmon. The start line was crowded as we looked for a place to stand. In the midst of the crowd, the frigid temperature wasn't as apparent as we huddled together.

"Maybe we can all run the whole race in a big crowd like this to conserve heat," Marilyn kidded. We were still laughing about her idea and jumping up and down to stay warm when the starting gun sounded. The crowd surged forward in the kind of closely packed group that Marilyn had imagined, but soon we were separated as I ran ahead.

The next day, a local newspaper published a photograph of the start of the race. In the photo, the runners are packed together in a group of several hundred. I'm in the middle of the photo sandwiched between several runners. Many are wearing wool hats and jackets to ward off the cold. I'm wearing gloves and a dark sweatshirt. I haven't seen them since. A doctor later told me the ambulance attendants had probably cut off the shirt in order to attach contact points to my chest as they strained to find a heartbeat. Marilyn is still next to me in the photo although I appear to be running slightly ahead of her. I didn't know it at the time, but just in front of me are two of the doctors who would later save my life.

The Harriers 8K, as the race is called, is a hilly course. It starts from the elevated fairgrounds hall, runs down a gravel roadway, and then turns onto a paved country road. The route meanders past farms and suburban homes and doubles back on itself twice so that competitors can see other runners both ahead and behind at different times. After completing registrations, Merrell walked out along the route to cheer on the runners at the halfway point where the route circles past the fairgrounds again. She saw me run by and thought that the race looked like a struggle for me. She assumed that I hadn't run in a while, and was just starting to train again.

In fact, I had been training hard for the race. I was looking forward to this year's nine-race series because of my increased training and remember feeling frustrated that my extra work hadn't been paying dividends. I was running more miles, but my body wasn't responding.

One memory I have of the race is seeing a frozen duck pond as we ran by one of the many small farms along the race route. The cold air would have been causing me to breathe hard. I like to start out strong when I race and then settle into a steady gait, often running behind or alongside someone who has a similar pace. But my eventual finishing time was almost two minutes slower than the time I had been expecting to finish. I must have been struggling. The cold air was probably hampering me. I probably felt frustrated by the other runners passing me along the route.

The final 100 metres of the course is a tough, uphill climb to the finish line. Rob Reid, a local running-store owner and friend, had finished earlier and was running back along the race route for a cool down as I neared the finish. He noticed me about 15 metres from the finish line. We ran by each other and did a "high-five," slapping each other's hand in a victory salute moments before I crossed the finish line.

The official race results show that I crossed the finish line at 34 minutes and 23 seconds. The end of these races is often a sprint, and I assume I was working hard to keep up with the runners around me. I came in beside another man in the 40s category and one second behind a woman from the University of Victoria running team. I've never found it easy to back down from a challenge at the end of these races. I was probably pushing myself, knowing that my time was slower than usual.

Immediately after crossing the finish line, my legs began to buckle. As I staggered toward the volunteer collecting race tags, she reached out to take my number off my race bib just as I collapsed into her. She later told me, "You died in my arms."

Do we experience anything when we die?

Running directly behind me was Ron Youngash, an emergency room physician. I fell right in front of him, gashing the side of my head, face, and arm on the frozen gravel road.

I'd never met any of the men and women who assisted me after the race. In fact, Ron and I didn't meet face-to-face, at least consciously, for several weeks. Ron's a person who's rarely without a grin on his face. But like all emergency medical professionals, he's quick to action when he's needed.

A young running-store clerk, Dan Baker, had also just arrived at the finish line when I collapsed. He quickly moved to my side to assist Ron. Dan was a recent university graduate who spent his summers working for the provincial parks system. He had taken some industrial first aid courses in conjunction with his parks work and knew how to perform Cardiopulmonary Resuscitation (CPR). He helped Ron try to figure out what had happened to me.

At first I was breathing but didn't respond to their questions.

I was bleeding from a cut on my forehead, and they weren't sure why I had fallen or what the problem was. They tried to comfort me, but my condition quickly deteriorated. Then I stopped breathing.

For the first time in my life, my heart had ceased to beat. The organ that sustains us – the pump that keeps blood circulating through our bodies, keeps oxygen flowing to our brains, maintains life in the furthest extremities of our limbs – no longer functioned.

My heart started beating while I was in my mother's womb. The heart of a fetus usually begins its pumping at 21 days. Mine had taken in oxygen-lacking blood, replenishing that blood with fresh oxygen, and pumping it back for over 40 years.

Now it had stopped. This was the end. The real finish line.

Is there such a thing as running too much or running too hard?

I knew many runners who seemed to thrive on pushing themselves to extremes. One man found the eight and 10 kilometre distances of the regular road races in Victoria not challenging enough, so he ran to the start of the races from his home. Sometimes he'd run 20 kilometres to get to the race, compete in the regular 10 kilometres, then immediately run the 20 kilometres back home. Several runners I knew trained every day, their morning 15 kilometres a pre-breakfast ritual.

Not all runners are that driven. I never considered myself to be an extreme runner. At least I didn't think I was. My pattern was to run three or four times each week for 40 minutes to an hour. I didn't try to push myself hard, but I did keep track of how far and how fast I'd run. During the race itself, I had started out with Marilyn, but quickly set out on my own, finding her pace too slow. Runners think like that. We may train in groups, but when it comes to races, we're individuals competing with ourselves and against those whose abilities are close to ours.

There was nothing wrong with thinking that way, I believed. Yet frequently, a nagging feeling would permeate my consciousness when I ran. Like most runners, I often thought about how much I should be pushing my body. The cautionary tale often cited about runners competing to extremes is the story of Jim Fixx. The author of the bestselling guide, *The Complete Book of Running*, Fixx became internationally famous for promoting the increased life expectancy resulting from regular physical exercise. His death from a heart attack at the age of 52 immediately following his daily run became fodder for comedians and justification for couch potatoes everywhere. For many runners, though, Fixx's death is never far from our minds. If this could happen to him, why couldn't it happen to me?

As I lay on the gravel roadway, directly beneath the finish line banner spanning the road, dozens of runners passed me in their sprints to the finish. Many checked their watches as they crossed the line, most gasped for breath having pushed to better their times, and all became at least subtly aware of their own mortality as they glanced down, thankful they hadn't succumbed like Jim Fixx and, as it appeared to be, like me.

2

FLATLINED

"Check his pulse." Ron, the ER doctor, had immediately taken charge.

"My fingers are so cold, I can't tell if he has one," Dan told Ron.

Ron leaned over, trying to listen to my breath. "He's not breathing."

"Should I start CPR?"

"Quickly."

With the other runners finishing the race around them, Ron initiated mouth-to-mouth resuscitation and Dan began chest compressions.

CPR is designed to keep a victim's heart and brain supplied with blood and oxygen after the heart stops beating and until medical help arrives. It involves two major techniques: chest compressions and ventilation, or mouth-to-mouth resuscitation. Chest compressions are used when the heart is stopped or in a state of ventricular fibrillation (the lower chambers of the heart twitching randomly and ineffectively). Chaotic fibrillation prevents the heart from contracting properly and thus pumping blood. The chest compressions keep the heart fibrillating, so it won't cease movement entirely, and pushes a limited amount of blood through the blood stream.

Ventilation keeps oxygen in the blood flowing to the brain. Once someone stops breathing, the oxygen content of the blood plummets. Brain cells stop functioning very quickly after oxygen has been cut off. Four to six minutes after breathing has stopped, brain damage is possible. Between six to 10 minutes, brain damage is likely. When a patient is without oxygen for over 10 minutes, irreversible brain damage is certain.

Soon after Ron and Dan started CPR, I vomited. Ron turned me on my side to clear an air passage. They were monitoring my condition when Cheryl Wood arrived on the scene. Cheryl is a retired anesthetist. When I finally met her weeks later, I was surprised to see a vibrant, fit, fifty-something woman, hardly the retired physician I'd expected. Like Ron, she's a take-charge individual. Cheryl had finished the race and was in the change room when someone ran in looking for a blanket to bring out to me. Cheryl ran back outside to see if she could help.

I was unconscious and my breathing shallow when Cheryl got there. She tried to take my pulse, but because I was so cold and because her fingers were numb, she was unable to determine the strength of my pulse. Then it became obvious that I was in real trouble. As an anesthetist, Cheryl can recognize when someone is in danger. My breathing stopped entirely for the second time and my skin started to turn a pasty grey colour. Cheryl began chest compressions again.

By then, many people had gathered around. Just finishing the run and wondering what had happened, Rachel Staples, a dentist, pushed her way through the crowd. Without hesitation, she knelt beside Cheryl and began mouth-to-mouth. Ron and Dan stayed close by, ready to spell off the two women if needed.

Can CPR really keep you alive?

The key to successful CPR is early intervention. Waiting even a few seconds to begin chest compressions and ventilation can mean the difference between the patient living and dying, and between having normal brain function and acute brain injury. When they started, Cheryl and Rachel had no idea that others had performed CPR on me already. They simply saw someone in distress and, as medical practitioners, knew they had no time to hesitate or ask questions.

Rachel and Cheryl estimated they performed CPR on me for 20 minutes. When I later asked them what kept them going for that long even though I had no signs of life the whole time they worked, Cheryl replied offhandedly, "We couldn't have stopped. You're too young."

Rachel is young herself. She has the slim build of an athlete and the self-assured nature of a doctor. When I met her and Cheryl together for the first time, Cheryl was surprised to learn that Rachel had never performed CPR in an emergency. She had only practised it during her dentistry training. "You're good at it," Cheryl told her at that meeting.

Other people around them offered to help, including Dan

and Ron who were still there, but they didn't need more than two people. As Rachel continued to breathe life into me, a runner passed an airway mask and a pair of latex gloves to her. He had been running in the race with them just in case of an emergency. Another runner, a friend of Cheryl's put his hand on Cheryl's shoulder and asked if he could pray for me. Cheryl smiled at him and said, "Go for it, Johnny."

An airline pilot, John Catterall was in his early thirties and avidly involved in running and church activities. His job as a pilot kept him ready to respond to unexpected situations. John later told me that he had almost not come to the race that day. In fact he had missed church to take part in the run, something he didn't like to do. But he felt compelled to attend the race. An elder in his church had told him recently that he would soon be presented with a profound opportunity to witness to his faith. On the way to the race that day, he prayed that this predicted opportunity would be revealed to him soon. When he saw me unconscious on the ground with his friend Cheryl pumping on my chest, he thought his prayers had already been answered.

He knelt beside Cheryl and took off the sweatshirt he'd been wearing in the run. He had forgotten that underneath the sweatshirt, he was wearing a bright red t-shirt with Jesus printed boldly across the chest. He was embarrassed, first by the shirt and second about the idea of praying so publicly for a man he didn't know. He was so compelled by the desire to do something and so moved by the synchronicity of events in his own life that had led to this moment, however, that he knew he had to start. With Cheryl's consent, John laid his hands on Cheryl and me and began to pray. John asked those standing around if anyone else would join him in praying for me as well. Four of them knelt beside me and quietly prayed with John.

Is prayer more powerful than paramedics?

The ambulance crew report records that a 911 call was received at 12:10 p.m. The first of two ambulances that were dispatched arrived at the scene at 12:22. Having finished the race in just over 34 minutes, I had crossed the finish line and collapsed 48 minutes earlier, at approximately 11:34.

When the ambulance arrived, Cheryl and Rachel in turn exchanged CPR functions with the paramedics. Finding no pulse, the ambulance crew used an ECG monitor to read my heart functions. The heart rhythm strip showed no heart activity at all. I was flatlined. Acting quickly, the paramedics set up a portable defibrillating machine, which would deliver an electrical charge to my heart in order to shock it back into a regular rhythm.

The attendants set the defibrillating machine to 200 watts, called for everyone to clear, and sent the electrical shock through my chest. My upper body immediately lurched upward with the shock. A faint blip appeared on the screen. Calling for all to clear a second time, they jolted my chest once more. Immediately, the ECG monitor showed a regular heart beat, my pulse returned, my blood pressure was recorded at 110/80, and the grey pallor in my face – the death mask as some medical practitioners call it – began to recede.

A second ambulance, used for advanced life support, then

arrived. One of the paramedics in the second ambulance started an intravenous drip and administered 80 mg. of lidocaine, a medication used to treat arrhythmias, in order to regulate my heartbeat. Placing a mask over my mouth and nose, the paramedics began a flow of oxygen in order to improve the amount getting to my brain. By now, the paramedics had lifted me onto a stretcher and wheeled my unconscious body into the ambulance. All those who had been helping to save my life for close to an hour by that point – putting blankets on my body still clad in thin running gear, placing hands on me in prayer, pumping rhythmically on my motionless chest, and breathing oxygen into my gaping mouth – watched as the ambulance sped away. Cheryl, still tired from her run and 20 minutes of vigorous chest compressions, turned to the others and shook her head.

"I don't think he's going to make it," she said.

Merrell was in charge of the presentation at the end of the race. Usually the gatherings after these races are a raucous blend of camaraderie and conversation. But Merrell remembered the subdued feeling in the hall that day as everyone gathered after the last runners had finished and the ambulances had left. While the more than 600 runners waited for the results to be tabulated, the race director phoned the hospital to check on my condition. Merrell announced to the waiting crowd that I was alive but still comatose. She felt helpless, but knew she had to do something. So she asked the runners to bow their heads for a minute and to collectively send positive energy to me.

At the end, Merrell called out, "Hang in there, Greg," and the crowd erupted in a cheer.

"The feeling was really amazing," Merrell told me later. "It almost took the roof off. It may not have helped as much as the CPR, but I know it helped some."

I have no memory of the ambulance ride. I was unconscious the entire time. The ambulance left the fairgrounds at 12:36, arriving at the Victoria General Hospital at 12:52. The fact that I was breathing at all is remarkable in itself. CPR is only effective when administered properly and promptly. If bystander CPR is not provided to a cardiac arrest victim, his chances of survival drop 7 to 10% for each minute of delay before defibrillation can be provided. Doctors surrounded me as I lay on that Saanichton roadside fighting for my life. They fought with me. As trained professionals, they knew how to respond in an emergency. They were responsible for the ambulance carrying a breathing man rather than a lifeless body.

I think of the ambulance ride often. Every time I see an ambulance racing down a street or hear sirens wailing by, I stop what I'm doing and try to remember. The sirens captivate me. I'm not trapped by them as Ulysses was by the calls of his mythical sirens, but I want them to help me. I want the sounds of the sirens to open the memories of that only ambulance ride I've ever taken. I'd like to be aware of the feeling of streaming down the highway, or pulling to a stop in front of the hospital, of being wheeled into the emergency room. I'd like to hear the ambulance attendants barking out my vital statistics as they pass the responsibility of my survival, of my life, to the emergency room physicians.

I've tried to remember all of the events of that day leading up to the ambulance ride. I've longed for some perspective on how I felt during the run, how hard I was pushing myself, and even some understanding of the pain I probably felt as my heart went into cardiac arrest. Sometimes I can recall a vague memory of slipping away, of losing consciousness, of drifting into an entirely different state all together. My memory is hazy, but the feeling is warm and compelling. I feel that all I need to do is keep running, keep moving in the direction of the warmth.

But the memory isn't clear and I'm not sure if it's a memory that I'm evoking myself or one that's truly part of my consciousness. Memory is rarely clear. It's shaped by time and new experiences, by pain and even joy. Some suggested that I couldn't retrieve the memory of my collapse because it was too difficult, too horrifying for me to recall. I was protecting myself by not remembering. In any case, it would be several days before any tangible, conscious memory would return.

3

A MAZE OF TUBES AND WIRES

"Hi, Debbie. It's Leslie."

"Hi, Leslie. What's up?"

"I'm sorry to be the one to tell you, but…."

"Tell me what?"

"It's Greg. He collapsed at the end of the race."

Since becoming a husband and father, I'd feared receiving a phone call that my wife or children had been injured. I'd often imagined myself staring in disbelief at the telephone receiver unable to comprehend the unexpected message. I'd pictured myself racing around the house in disarray trying to figure out what course of action to take. I'd felt the quiver of my voice phoning other loved ones to relate the news and ask for help. I'd only imagined all these events. But Debbie lived them.

At about 1 p.m. on January 11th, she received that phone call. It was from our neighbour, Leslie Hopkin. A friend of hers had been at the race and when she found out that I was the collapsed runner everyone was crowded around, she phoned Leslie asking her to tell Debbie. All she knew at the time was that I had collapsed, so Debbie was hopeful that I had simply succumbed to exhaustion, or the cold, and she accepted Leslie's offer of a ride to the hospital. Leslie's friend had told her that the ambulance was going to the Royal Jubilee Hospital, which is near our home, so Debbie and Leslie headed there.

Along the way, Leslie told Debbie a little more of the details she knew. For the first time, Debbie found out that I was unconscious and had stopped breathing. She knew nothing else. They arrived at the hospital and went straight to the emergency ward thinking they would have to wait for the ambulance to arrive. When Debbie told the receptionist she was waiting for an ambulance, the receptionist immediately tried contacting the attendants. That was when they found out that the ambulance had gone to the Victoria General Hospital instead, a 25-minute drive from there. The receptionist told Debbie that I was breathing again and that she should not rush to get to the hospital. But taking her time was not what Debbie had in mind. She asked Leslie to drop her off at her parents' house so she could get a ride to the hospital from her mother, Vi.

The Victoria General Hospital is located north of Victoria's city centre. It was built in 1983 and is situated just off the highway that runs up Vancouver Island. It backs onto a large wooded area giving it a rural atmosphere. The ample grounds have become the home to hundreds of rabbits that seem to have made the hospital grounds their own. Their lineage can probably be traced to a single pair abandoned by some ungrateful recipient of a live

Easter present. Their burgeoning numbers, their vibrant life, contrast starkly with the illness within the hospital.

Do we need permission to cry?

Vi dropped Debbie at the front door and drove off to find a parking spot while Debbie raced in. She approached the reception area just inside the door. The receptionist was looking at her computer when Debbie reached the counter.

"Excuse me," she said to the receptionist.

"Just a moment, please," she replied without looking up.

Debbie is not a pushy person, but she was in no mood to wait. "My husband was just brought in by ambulance. Could you tell me where he is?"

With a sharp glance at Debbie then back at her computer, the receptionist asked, "What is his name?" When Debbie told her my name, she typed it into the computer and watched the screen as some information came up that Debbie couldn't see.

She looked up at Debbie. "I'll need to get some information from you." Then she turned back to her computer. "How old is your husband?"

"He's 40."

"What is his height?"

Debbie tried to choke back her tears. "Uhh, almost six feet, I think."

"His weight?"

"His weight? I can't remember. I just need to know if he's okay."

"Do you have his Care Card?"

By this point Debbie was sobbing. "No, I don't have his Care Card. Can't you just tell me where he is?"

Finally the receptionist relented. "Well, just let me see what I can do," she told Debbie as she picked up the phone.

Soon, an attendant appeared and led Debbie and Vi, who had rushed in after parking the car, to a small room furnished with a couch, a chair, and a telephone. Debbie knew something must be terribly wrong when the attendant didn't take her to see me right away. After a few, long minutes, a doctor came into the room to talk to Debbie. By the solemn look on his face and the sombre tone of his voice, Debbie could tell the situation was serious. Bluntly, he began to explain my condition to her.

"Your husband is alive and breathing," he said, "but he's comatose and on life support. We're not sure when, or even if, he'll come out of the coma."

He admitted that he wasn't really sure how well I would be functioning if I did revive since I had been without oxygen for so long. He didn't know whether I would be able to breathe on my own and whether I would ever be able to talk or walk or write or have any memory at all.

Debbie broke into tears of disbelief. She didn't know how this disaster could so suddenly occur, how I could possibly be in such a state.

As Debbie wept, the doctor put his hand on her shoulder and said, "It's all right if you cry. I expect you to cry."

Debbie was incredulous. "You expect me to cry?" she said. "You're giving me permission to cry?" Her tears became angry, frustrated sobs.

"I'm sorry," the doctor said awkwardly trying to comfort her.

Through her tears, Debbie asked the doctor whether he thought she should call my parents in Calgary, Alberta, to tell them what had happened. Without hesitating, he nodded his head. So Debbie called my sister, Luanne, who lives in Saanichton, to tell her what had happened and to ask her to call my parents.

Where did I go?

Finally, Debbie was taken into the emergency room to see me. I was lying on a stretcher, unconscious, with a maze of tubes and wires running from my body to various machines. The emergency report written about me states that, because I had no airway control and was both hyperventilating and underbreathing, I had been intubated in the ambulance and placed on a respirator that breathed for me. Debbie's first reaction was that I didn't look like myself at all.

"I just kept wondering where he was," Debbie remembered, "where his mind was, what was happening inside him. I kept thinking that I wasn't really looking at him, that it was some movie or something that was really unreal."

People frequently ask me if I drifted into an out-of-body state, seeing my own body from above, as I lay comatose on the hospital gurney. They wonder if I glimpsed the mythical light at the end of the tunnel that some people who've gone through near-death experiences have written and talked about. I was near death certainly. In fact, for twenty minutes I had been clinically dead. But

I have no memory of glimpsing a light or viewing myself from above. In a way, I feel almost removed from the whole event. I was experiencing the coma, but I can't remember it. Those who waited desperately at my side have the fuller experience of my coma.

I often wonder about descriptions of out-of-body experiences and metaphysical visions, especially those depicted in films. When I've read the work of people who've tried to write about mystical experiences, they often describe them as inexplicable. Is the mystical explicable? Can we really see as clearly in our minds as we can with our eyes? Of course, filmmakers are forced to make visual that which is often without visual form.

I've tried to remember what I felt or saw while comatose. I've searched for some kind of explanation of why the events of January 11th occurred and why they happened to me. I've longed to find answers.

But the more I've tried, the more distant those answers have become. Ironically, just as when I would finally stop running from the fears I perceived in my childhood nightmares in order to let go of them, the less I tried to find answers, see truths, or long for visions, the more I began to feel, sense, understand, and actually see.

4

COMATOSE

"I just can't believe this could have happened," Debbie said to Rob Reid, the running-store owner who'd been at the race. "Did you see Greg during the run?"

"Yes, I talked to him before the race, and then I saw him again just before he finished. I even congratulated him as he was running up the final hill. But I didn't see the end."

"How did he look when you saw him?"

"He was smiling. He looked fine."

Knowing that I was at least stable, Debbie had returned home to attend to our three children – Lucas, 15, Raechel, 12, and Leo, 5 – and prepare to come back to the hospital for the night. She arrived at our house to find Rob sitting at the kitchen table playing a board game with the kids. He had come straight from the race to see if he could help.

Even then, at the age of 43, Rob was still one of the best long distance runners in the country, ranked in the top 10 in the marathon. We'd been friends since I wrote a magazine profile about him several years earlier. We're both tall and slim with curly red hair, so we're often confused for one another. In fact, many people thought it was Rob being attended to at the race and were shocked to see him walking around after the ambulance had left. When he heard that people thought he had collapsed, he knew instantly that I was the one who had been taken away in the ambulance. So he immediately drove to our house.

Debbie later said she was surprised to see Rob begin to cry as he talked to her and realized that things were so serious. He volunteered to drive Debbie back to the hospital after she arranged for the children and packed a bag for herself and one for me. Driving back to the hospital with Rob, Debbie was still dumbfounded about the whole situation.

Looking out the window of Rob's car, she began to cry. "He looked so awful at the hospital, Rob. All those tubes."

Rob didn't know what to say. "Maybe he'll seem better when you get back there."

"I don't know. I don't know if I even want to see him. I mean I want to see him. I'm just so scared. I don't know what it's going to be like."

Can you hear anything when you're in a coma?

By the time Debbie arrived back at the hospital, I had been moved to the coronary care unit (CCU). Debbie met my sister, Luanne, and my brother-in-law, Keith, in the waiting room adjacent to the CCU. Luanne is 18 months younger than I am. All our lives, we've been close, and that relationship has spread to our spouses as well.

I consider Keith one of my best friends, and Debbie feels the same way about Luanne. Keith and Luanne live minutes away from the Saanichton Fairgrounds where the race began and ended. The race route actually runs within sight of their home. In fact, I had planned to visit Luanne after the race. She had coffee prepared and was waiting for me when Debbie called to tell her what had happened.

When the nurse on duty finally came to take Debbie to my room to see me, Debbie asked if Luanne could come in as well. My condition hadn't changed. I was still unconscious, covered with tubes and surrounded by beeping and blinking machines. The nurse encouraged Debbie and Luanne to sit with me as long as they wanted. "Even though he's in a coma, he's still aware," she told them. "He knows you're here. Go ahead. Talk to him. Touch him."

Debbie and Luanne held my hands, told me that they loved me and reassured me that everything was going to be okay. My body twitched frequently, so Debbie massaged my legs and feet. They thought the twitching was a result of my not having cooled down after the run.

Luanne was impressed with the care I received in those first few hours. She said that the nurses on my shift never went to the nursing station, staying the whole shift in the room with me. At the time, they believed that I had received CPR for ten minutes. They kept telling Debbie and Luanne that being without oxygen and not breathing for ten minutes was a long time. Luanne realized the nurses were gently trying to tell them that, when I did come to, I might be suffering from brain damage. When they later found out that I had been oxygen deprived for 20 minutes, their fears were compounded.

Debbie asked one of the doctors who came in to check on me whether she should have the children come up to see me. He agreed it would be a good idea since they didn't know when or if I would wake up.

How can you prepare children for death?

Vi brought the children up that evening. They were ushered into the CCU waiting room. By that time, my family had virtually taken over the room. Luanne tried to prepare the three of them for seeing me.

"When I take you into the room," she told them, "your dad will look like he's asleep. In fact he is asleep. He just can't wake up yet." She reached out to hold Raechel's hand. "The tubes you'll see in his nose and the wires attached to his body look scary, but they're helping him breathe and helping the doctors to understand what's going on in your dad's body. So don't be frightened. You can talk to him. He can probably hear you."

They then went into my room to join Debbie.

Leo walked right up to my bedside looking at the wires and monitors. "Guess what, Dad," he said without hesitation. "We had bagels for lunch today." He looked across at the serious faces of his family members and then at the wires and tubes on my body. "It's going to be okay. I saw all of this on Mr. Rogers once."

Lucas tentatively touched my unmoving arm and said, "I know you'll come through this, Dad."

Raechel had remained close to the door. She wasn't sure what to do. To her, I looked asleep, but not entirely there with them. She walked to the side of my bed, kissed my forehead, and said, "I love you, Daddy."

When they returned to the waiting room, Lucas and Raechel both started to cry. Through her tears, Raechel asked, "What happened to his face?" While preparing them for the shock of the tubes and monitors, Luanne had forgotten to explain that I had hit my head and scraped my face when I fell at the end of the race. The look of it shocked Raechel.

It's difficult for me to imagine what my family members were thinking as they gathered at my bedside and in the adjacent waiting room while I lay in a coma. Brain damage seemed inevitable even if I did emerge from the coma. They couldn't believe this had happened to me. A forty-year-old runner wasn't supposed to have a cardiac arrest. Their husband, father, and brother was supposed to help with balancing the cheque book, going over homework, and caring for aging parents, not suffer brain damage.

As five-year-old Leo looked around the room at his gathered, emotional relatives, he looked puzzled. "Why is everyone crying?" he asked.

The laughter that came as a response to his simple but genuine question was a relief for everyone. In fact, the tension of the next few weeks was often broken by Leo's direct, immediate needs.

My family has always delighted in children. They've never been the types to feel overwhelmed by children's demands, distracted by their concerns, or frustrated by their cries. I remember my grandfather telling a story about having lunch in a restaurant one day. He was on his own, enjoying a peaceful break from the pressures of his printing business. The only other patrons of the restaurant were a young couple and their child. For much of the meal, the child fussed and cried. As my grandfather was leaving, he had to walk past the family's table. Both parents looked up at him and apologized for the noise of their little boy.

My grandfather stopped them. "There's no need to apologize," he said. "I have six children and 16 grandchildren and I've heard all of them cry many times. There's only one grandchild I didn't hear. And I would give anything to have heard that boy cry."

My aunt and uncle's first child was stillborn. His birth cries never came. Years later, my grandfather still mourned that loss. Like my family and like me, he loved children. He saw in them the promise of hope and the spark of the Divine.

Leo emanated that as well. While my family waited in the hospital, his simple, childlike concerns helped everyone else realize that there was a world beyond the hospital rooms they would inhabit for the next several days. Keeping him close was important. He embodied life and future as I lay clinging to life, my future uncertain.

5

A GLASGOW COMA SCORE
CAN GO NO LOWER THAN THREE

"I know this is difficult for you, Debbie," our family doctor, Nick Fairhurst, said warmly. "This is the worst thing anyone could imagine happening."

When Dr. Fairhurst entered the Intensive Care Unit of the Victoria General Hospital at 8 o'clock the morning after the race, he must have already heard about my condition. Instead of going into the room where I lay comatose, intubated, and monitored constantly, he had walked straight toward Debbie in the waiting room, taken her arm, and gently led her away from the family gathered around her so he could talk to her alone.

"I know you want to do what's right for Greg, but you've got to take care of yourself as well," he told her. "Greg is getting the best care he could possibly receive here. And the only way you can help him is by being rested and well yourself."

Debbie collapsed in a flood of tears on his shoulder.

Dr. Nick Fairhurst had been our family doctor for over 15

years. He delivered our daughter Raechel and our younger son Leo. His children attended the school where I taught. Lucas and his daughter were friends in elementary school even going to each other's birthday parties. I'd watched Nick referee rugby matches. And I'd watched his son play rugby for the Canadian national team. We always ended any medical visit with a friendly chat about our children.

But Debbie was his patient too, and he knew he had to care for her even before he took a look at me. By that point, Debbie needed his support. She hadn't slept that night.

The first night was difficult for my family as they waited at my bedside. Several doctors had examined me after my arrival. Their reports, written that evening, offered little hope for my recovery. A neurologist suggested that I might have suffered "significant anoxic brain injury" after having been deprived of adequate oxygen for so long. Another doctor wrote, "Unfortunately at this point, he is comatose and thus his survival and recovery are very guarded."

Prior to 1974, the only way for medical practitioners to describe the extent of a patient's coma was descriptive. They would use vague terms such as lethargic, stuporous, or semi-conscious. The problem was the terms were not objective. One doctor's lethargic might be another's stuporous.

In 1974, two neurosurgeons in Glasgow, Scotland, Drs. Teasdale and Jennett, developed a standard for quantifying the level of consciousness of patients. They produced what has become known as the Glasgow Coma Score (GCS). Medical observers can determine a patient's consciousness level by recording the individual's best eye response, verbal response, and motor response. The patient's responses are graded 1 to 4 for eye response and 1 to 5 for verbal and motor responses with 1 meaning no response at all. The scores are totaled to give an indication of the severity of the potential brain injury. The possible brain injury is described as Minor if the GCS is 13-15, Moderate if the GCS is 9-12, or Severe if the GCS is 8 or under.

According to the paramedics' report, my response was rated 1 in every category. My GCS score was 3. The state of my coma was profound and the extent of the brain injury I'd received by being deprived of oxygen was likely severe. I remained in that state throughout the night.

How does a parent feel seeing a child near death?

At about 10:30 that night, my parents arrived from Calgary. They had been able to catch a flight almost immediately after hearing about my collapse and were brought to the hospital by two of our friends. Other friends had gathered at the hospital after hearing the news. One, who had been at the race, arrived early in the evening with two bags of food and drink for my family. The members of a men's group I belong to, met in the hospital cafeteria and, from four floors below my room, stayed long into the night sending prayers and positive energy my way.

Debbie, my mother, Luanne, and Lucas all stayed in my room that night. I was heavily sedated with morphine, still intubated, and breathing with the help of a ventilator. Luanne later described the night as "surreal" and "haunting." The four of them sat in various positions around my bed keeping track of the constantly beeping and blinking monitors.

At some point in the night, I started to stir. Not wanting me to come out of the coma in the middle of the night or damage my throat struggling against the tube that was allowing me to breath, the doctors kept me sedated. Every hour and a half, a nurse would come into my room and administer another dose of morphine through my intravenous drip.

What does a physician really mean describing a patient's recovery as guarded?

My family maintained a vigil at my bedside throughout the next morning. I remained intubated and heavily medicated. Doctors continued to describe my condition as serious and guarded. My parents considered having my two sisters in Calgary fly to Victoria as well, fearing they'd never see me alive again.

The waiting for my family was painful. They had been given scanty information about my condition because the doctors knew very little. They had no idea why a healthy man would collapse with a cardiac arrest at the end of a running race. They talked about a sudden death event, a catchall description for any unexplained death. I was still alive, but I hovered near death all that morning. They asked my parents about illnesses when I was a child. They asked Debbie about my health in the last few months. None of the information they received suggested a reason for my collapse. They simply had to wait, to see how I would respond over the next few hours.

That afternoon, after almost an entire day of giving me doses of morphine every hour and a half, the hospital staff felt it was time to take a step toward encouraging my recovery by removing the breathing tube and taking me off the ventilator to see if I would be able to breathe on my own. A young respirologist came into the room and asked my family to wait out in the hall as he took the tube out. This was an important step. I hadn't yet emerged from the coma and I was still heavily sedated. If I were able to breathe without the help of a ventilator, my chances of survival would be much greater.

From the hallway, my family could hear the respirologist at work. They heard a slight gurgling sound as he slowly pulled out the tube. Then they heard nothing. Soon, they heard the voice of the respirologist. He was shouting.

"Richard. Breathe! Come on, Richard. You can breathe!"

My family grew more tense the longer the respirologist kept up his efforts. My sister, Luanne, tried to break the tension. "Whoever this Richard guy is, he must be having trouble breathing as well."

My family laughed nervously until they heard the respirologist again. "Come on, Richard!"

By then, my mother had had enough. From the hallway she angrily called back into the room, "His name's Greg, not Richard."

Debbie reached over and put her hand on my mom's shoulder. "It's okay," she told her. "We know."

Finally, after several minutes of shouting from both inside and outside of the room, the respirologist opened the door. "You can come in now," he told my family.

Tentatively, my family entered my room. I lay on my back, still unconscious, but with no breathing tubes attached to me.

Nothing is more natural than breathing. We rarely think about it. As a runner, I was perhaps more aware of my breathing than most. To increase my air intake as I ran, I often tried to breathe in and out through my nose exclusively as a coach had once taught me. I never seemed to get enough oxygen via nose breathing, however, and would usually revert to open-mouthed gasping as I ran. Maybe I was running too hard. Perhaps I should have pushed my breathing only to the point where I could easily breathe through my nose.

But the deep breathing brought on by a run always invigorated me. I'd feel cleansed after a run, my lungs pulsating with the vigour of replenished oxygen. What is more of a sign of life than breath itself?

When the paramedics intubated me in order to regulate my breathing, they were trying to regulate my life. But they were doing so artificially. When the respirologist removed the breathing tube, he was eliminating the artificial and reintroducing the normal – giving back to me the most important bodily function we possess. Breathing is life. Removing a breathing tube takes a patient in one of two directions. As my lungs filled on their own, with no breathing tube, with no external pumps, I had unconsciously begun my journey back to life.

6

WAITING AND PRAYING

"We're at the point now where we have to consider Greg's neurological state if and when he comes out of the coma," a neurologist told my family after the breathing tube was removed. "Unfortunately, oxygen deprivation can cause serious brain damage. The fact that his heart stopped beating for 20 minutes is not good."

Anoxic brain injury occurs when the brain does not receive oxygen. Because brain cells need oxygen to survive and function, they can quickly become impaired when the oxygen supply is cut off. The CPR I received allowed some oxygen to get to my brain. But the doctors in the hospital had no way of determining the extent to which that oxygen had been delivered.

"Yet there's always hope," the neurologist continued. "Everyday, people emerge from profound coma states with very little change in their brain functions. If Greg can follow you with his eyes when he wakes up, that will be a good sign. All we can do now is simply wait."

How much of your brain is damaged
after 20 minutes without a pulse?

My family could do little more than simply wait as I lay in my hospital bed, breathing on my own but still unconscious. As the nurses reduced the morphine they were administering me, I began to move more frequently and even make noises. None of the sounds coming out of my mouth were coherent, though, and my movements were jerky and spasmodic. My family watched every twitch and listened to every utterance hoping that something would make sense to them, that a sound would be a choked word of greeting or a gesture would indicate some attempt at communication.

The frequent visits from doctors and the almost constant attention from nurses in the 24 hours that I had been in the hospital had offered little hope for my family. Debbie had entered my room soon after my admission to find the two nurses who had been caring for me both crying. She looked at them dumbfounded and burst into tears herself as the three of them hugged beside my unconscious body.

The neurologist's comment about watching to see if I could follow them with my eyes hadn't reassured my family. They couldn't imagine what a bad sign would be if a simple eye movement was good. The neurologist was right about one thing. All they could do was wait.

And pray.

Does prayer really work?

I was raised a Roman Catholic and attended Catholic schools in Calgary throughout my schooling. For me, being Catholic was like having curly hair. There wasn't much I could do about it, so I just accepted it. I was an altar boy, I learned Latin phrases by rote so that I could respond to the prayers led by the priest, and I went to mass every week and confession once a month. I knelt by the side of my bed to pray every night until I was a teenager. I joined my family in saying the rosary together when we traveled to Saskatchewan to visit relatives once or twice a year. Because I attended a Catholic school, most of my friends were Catholic. I wore my Catholicism like a well-used jean jacket, not a hair shirt.

When I was 19, I spent seven months backpacking through Europe. As did most of the thousands of other young people traveling around Europe in the mid 1970s, I stayed at the requisite youth hostels, followed up on the freebies highlighted in the Europe-on-a-budget guides, and visited almost as many museums as pubs and bars. But I also stopped in at churches and cathedrals in every city I visited. Just before I left Canada, I had found out that my favourite uncle had been diagnosed with cancer. Denis was only ten years older that I was, and his illness was a blow to our whole family. Visiting all those churches held a purpose for me. In every one, I lit a candle and said a prayer for my uncle.

If the Catholic Church really wants to help the poor, why is it so rich?

With Denis in mind and after years of sermons and Catholic education, I made plans to travel to Rome. I considered my visit to Rome and the Vatican as almost a pilgrimage. I suppose I had expected some sort of spiritual awakening or mystical revelation when I disembarked from the train in Rome. But I was shocked by what confronted me. Rome was simply another huge city. And unlike other cities I had visited, it lacked some sort of salvaging characteristic. It didn't have the beauty of the canals in Venice, or the romance of the Latin Quarter in Paris, or the excitement of the theatre district in London.

Before I visited the Vatican, I toured the Roman ruins just outside Vatican City. Walking through the remains of the Coliseum, I learned that many of the missing stones from this ancient structure had been pilfered to use in the construction of St. Peter's Basilica. Why had I never heard of that? The Catholic Church had systematically plundered an ancient Roman edifice to create its most important ecclesiastical structure. That seemed wrong to my 19-year old conscience.

Then, when I finally did visit the Vatican and that imposing Basilica, an unexpected feeling overwhelmed me again. Yes, St. Peter's was stunning. Yes, the Sistine Chapel was one of the most awe-inspiring works of art I had witnessed. Yes, the Swiss guards presented great photo opportunities. But those observations were all part of the problem that was confronting me. My visit to Vatican City was not the culmination of the spiritual pilgrimage I had anticipated. All I could think of was the opulence, the money tied up in these works of art, the security needed to guard it, and the poverty just outside its gates.

Visiting Rome did change me, but not in the way I had expected. I began to question Catholicism for perhaps the first time in my life. I still felt connected to the spiritual aspects of the faith, but its temporal concerns bothered me. I didn't stop visiting Catholic churches throughout Europe, though. When I returned home to Canada, I continued to go to church. When I moved to Victoria to attend university, I joined a Catholic student organization.

And in Victoria I met Debbie. Debbie's religious affiliation had little to do with our relationship initially. She was raised an Anglican, but didn't consider herself part of that faith. In fact, as a teenager, she had become more involved in an evangelical religion that appealed to young people. As our relationship developed, she attended university masses with me. In fact, the chaplain of the university, Father Leo Robert, became a good friend who officiated at our wedding. He later baptized two of our children and we named our third after him. His death from cancer in 1990 saddened us deeply. Without the stability of a trusted mentor, we slowly began to drift away from the Catholic Church.

Is there a difference
between spirituality and religion?

After Raechel's birth, we started to look around for another church. Less than a block from our home we found a church that was, if not anything else, convenient. It was a United Church, part of neither Debbie's tradition nor mine. We started to attend services there and soon became friends with the young, student minister who was completing an internship at the church. Paul Taylor worked at the church for two summers. We kept in contact with him when he moved to Alberta to work as a minister there and were thrilled when he eventually returned to Victoria to work at a different United Church. He had returned to Victoria not long before my cardiac arrest. So he was one of the first people that Debbie called after my collapse.

The cold, clear weather of race day had turned to an unexpected snowfall the next day. Snow is so rare in Victoria that longtime residents refuse to venture out of their homes at the first sign of any snowfall accumulation. But Paul had spent the last several years in Alberta, so he wasn't impeded by a little snow. He convinced Kate, his new girlfriend who was later to become his wife, to drive him to the Victoria General to be with my family.

When he arrived, my family was continuing to hold vigil around my hospital bed, waiting for me to emerge from my unconscious state. He entered quietly and hugged Debbie who introduced him to my parents and my sister. Paul has the enthusiasm of a young idealist but the wisdom of a true spiritual scholar. The youngest person in the room, he immediately took charge and asked for everyone to hold hands. They stood in a circle with Paul at the foot of the bed, Debbie holding one of my hands, and my sister, Luanne, holding the other. Paul began to pray. As he prayed with his eyes closed, Luanne joined in but continued to look at me. She told me later that, as soon as Paul started to pray, I began to stir. Moments after he began, I opened my eyes. I didn't look

around at the others circling my bed and holding hands, but gazed
intently at Paul the whole time he spoke. As soon as Paul stopped,
I smiled at him and said, "Thank you for that, Paul," and closed
my eyes. Paul describes that moment as one of the most spiritual
experiences of his life.

For many, spirituality and religion are synonymous. Yet people not
wanting to link themselves with religious extremism will say, "I'm
spiritual, but not religious," often without truly knowing what
they mean. When I found myself conflicted over the opulence of a
church that had been an enormous part of my life, I was grappling
with the difference between spirituality and religion.

But we don't need to look to religious institutions to find
spirituality. To be sure, some do find Spirit in the great cathedrals
of the world or even the simple country churches in isolated vil-
lages. But for others, Spirit resides in the call of a loon or the roar
of an ocean tide. I believe we can find the spiritual in the everyday occurrence: in the laugh of a child or the majesty of a soaring
eagle, in the emotion of an opera aria or the geometric symmetry
of a Norfolk Pine tree. I think it's important to see the spiritual in
the ordinary. If we rely on towering gothic spires or centuries of
theological dogma to define what most deeply touches us, we can
miss the depth of Spirit occurring all around us everyday.

In his poem, "Ode to a Nightingale," John Keats explored the
real spirituality he felt in the simple birdsong that for him was
truly immortal when he wrote, "The voice I hear this passing night
was heard / In ancient days by emperor and clown." The call of
the nightingale that made him feel as though he had "emptied

some dull opiate to the drains," was as profound and timeless as the grandeur of any cathedral or the teachings of any religion. Just as Keats seems to suggest in his poem, I believe the spiritual is present everywhere and in every time.

As Paul led the prayer for me that evening and as a man who made his living practising and cultivating religion, he was well aware of the presence of Spirit. His prayer was based on a religious tradition and came from years of religious study and implementation, but the manifestation of his prayer was a spiritual moment centred on the depth of emotion everyone in that hospital room felt. I may not have suddenly emerged from my coma during the prayer, but those were the first coherent words that I had spoken. And they gave hope to everyone holding hands around that hospital bed.

7

THE INVINCIBILITY
OF THE RUNNER

"I've been looking after heart patients for almost 20 years," a nurse caring for me told my sister. "Most of them are overweight and out of shape. But your brother doesn't have an ounce of fat on his body."

"He's always been like that," Luanne replied.

"Really?"

"That's right. He was always skinny. And he was always running."

"Is there anything from his past that might have contributed to his cardiac arrest?"

"I can't think of anything."

How could someone
with no risk factors have heart disease?

As I slowly began to emerge from my coma, the doctors and nurses attending me in the hospital continued to question my family about my past to determine if I had any of the risk factors for heart disease. I was a 40-year-old male, which was a risk factor in itself. But I had no family history of heart disease. My grandfather had a pacemaker inserted in his chest late in his life, but he'd had no heart problems before then.

I'd never smoked. I had no obvious problems with cholesterol. I had left a fairly stressful job six years earlier and was now pursuing a desire to write for a living. I was trying to lead a balanced life and was proud of the fact that I was fit and slim.

Most of my fitness came from running. I'd always run. As a kid, I'd run home from school every day, often kicking a tin can down the alleys behind the houses along my route to amuse myself. In school I was known as a runner. I wasn't very big, but even the tallest, most athletic looking boys in my grade couldn't beat me when we were forced to endure timed runs in elementary school.

When it came time to compete in sports in junior high school, my speed and endurance kept me on the school teams. I was never the best, but I was usually the fastest. I ran to altar boy practice, I ran to Boy Scout meetings, and I ran just to have fun.

As a young adult, running became my preferred method for staying fit. When I traveled through Europe in my late teens, I remember going for a run through the streets of Aix-en-Provence in southern France the morning after I first arrived in Europe. Along the winding roads, I maneuvered around groups of school boys in short pants wearing leather satchels on their backs and carrying soccer balls under their arms, passed outdoor cafes where men sat smoking cigarettes and sipping espresso, and dodged winding moped riders leaving trails of blue exhaust with the distinct smell of oil mixed with gasoline. No one else was running. And almost everyone I passed looked at me in bemused puzzlement.

I ran my way around Europe and continued to run when I eventually moved to Victoria for university. The city was a perfect place to run. Unlike in Calgary, I could run outside in Victoria year round. The trails around the University of Victoria, the Dallas Road waterfront, even the winding streets of the out-of-the-way neighbourhoods that reminded me so much of Europe became my many and varied running routes.

Not until I was in my 30s did I begin to run in races. My son, Lucas, was the catalyst for that development. The year he was in grade 4, we both started September at home instead of in a school building. I had taken a leave from my teaching job to stay home and write. He was in the process of moving from the school where I had been teaching and he had attended, to the school where Raechel had just started kindergarten. There was no room for him in the school, temporarily, so I taught him at home for the first two months. We both loved it. I would write while he worked on math problems, kept a journal, and researched any science or social studies issue that interested him. Our lunches became home economics projects, and our PE classes were long runs. The weather was glorious that autumn so the runs were the highlight of our days. We decided on a goal to take part in the Terry Fox Run in late September. Running in memory of Terry Fox and his fight to end cancer was moving, and running with my 9-year-old son made the experience even more emotional.

Despite being home schooled at the beginning of the year, Lucas was still able to compete in the school district cross-country races. He won every race that year. His achievements spurred me on, and I started to run in some community races as well. The Victoria road-racing season extends for several months, so I had dozens of races to choose from. Running in races, often with Lucas but sometimes on my own, became a welcomed routine.

I was never able to win the ribbons and trophies that Lucas began to accumulate, but running for me that year wasn't about ribbons or trophies. It was about the camaraderie Lucas and I shared. And it was about what I believed was the steady, strong, solid beating of my heart.

Do runners ignore warning signs about their health more than non-runners?

The year I turned 40, I decided to run in the Royal Victoria Marathon 10K. I'd run it in the past and liked the atmosphere of the marathon that spilled over into the shorter route as well. The race took place two weeks before my birthday. My plan was to try running it in under 40 minutes, the symmetry of 40 years and 40 minutes appealing to me. It was a rainy, cool morning, just right for marathoners. But the race didn't feel right for me. I struggled across the finish line at 41 minutes and 15 seconds and immediately vomited: right in front of the legislative buildings, at the end of the long chute leading to the finish line, with hundreds of people lining the sidewalk watching. I was so embarrassed that I didn't even stop to consider what had caused me to be sick.

Had I thought about it, I might have done something. I might have gone for a check up with my doctor. I might have tried to slow down the pace of my running or abandoned the arbitrary finish times I had begun to aim for. At 40, I still felt and looked young and healthy. I had no reason to believe that I should be considering possible problems within my body. I felt as invincible as a teenager. And like most runners, I simply put up with the occasional stiff knees and swollen feet or even twinges in my chest that to me were inevitable and normal. But struggling across the finish line of a race only to lose my breakfast was not normal. Nor, unfortunately, was my ignoring of an obvious sign.

8

THE PRESENT
IS ALL WE'VE GOT

"Good morning, Greg. Do you know who this is?" a nurse asked pointing to Luanne, Debbie waiting anxiously on the other side of the bed.

After greeting Paul Taylor during his prayer the night before, I had immediately closed my eyes and passed a second night in a sedated but fitful sleep. Debbie, Luanne, and Lucas had spent that second night in the hospital as well, sleeping much less than I did. But as the light of morning began to fill my hospital room and my family watched my every movement, I began to stir more frequently. Remembering what the neurologist had said about my eye movement being a good sign of brain activity, they stared hopefully each time my eyes flickered.

Finally, the flickering movement stopped and my eyes stayed open. Luanne stood on one side of the bed beside the nurse who was leaning over me. Debbie stood on the other side of the bed.

"Do you know who this is?" the nurse asked again.

They all waited as I lay in the bed staring at my sister. "It's Luanne, of course," I said matter of factly. The three of them gasped and then laughed in excitement, almost jumping up and down.

From the other side of the bed, Debbie lurched forward, hugged me, and began covering my forehead and face with kisses. "I can't believe it," she said. "I just can't believe it."

I hugged her back, then, as she pulled away said, "Who are you?" Debbie was stunned. She looked across to Luanne, then back to me her face a mask of concern. When I smiled and said, "Hi, Debbie," she started kissing me again telling me how much she loved me.

They were elated. For the past 36 hours, they had maintained an unrelenting vigil at my bedside wondering if I would wake up and worrying about my state of mind if I did wake up. Debbie's imagination had run the gamut from life without me entirely to life with me in a vegetative state or life with me severely brain damaged. Now here I was, awake, and actually joking with her.

Their elation was soon tempered, though, when I began to speak more.

"Where are we?" I asked.

"We're in the hospital," Debbie answered.

"Why are we in the hospital?"

"You're in the hospital, Greg. You fell at the end of a race."

I looked around the room, confused. I glanced down at my hospital bracelet and looked up at Debbie.

"Why are we in the hospital?" I asked again.

Debbie paused. "I just told you, Greg. We're visiting you in the hospital."

"What happened to my hand?"

"You fell at the end of a race and scraped it."

"Well, let's go home," I said trying to get out of bed.

The nurse leaned over and held my shoulders, gently pushing me back against the pillow. "No, Greg. You have to stay still. You're still connected to all this equipment."

I looked down at the leads on my chest connected to a heart monitor and the tube in my arm connected to an IV bag dangling on a pole beside me.

"Why are we in the hospital?"

Debbie and Luanne both looked at the nurse. She took Debbie by the arm and moved to the other side of the room away from my bed while Luanne stayed beside me in case I needed to be restrained again.

"Don't worry, Debbie," she said. "It looks like he has a little short-term memory loss. It's not that unusual for patients coming out of a coma. It's probably just a temporary thing. Try to keep answering his questions without looking concerned."

Is lack of memory a sign of brain damage?

For the next hour, Debbie and Luanne did just that. Every time I asked a question, they'd calmly answer it. When I asked the same question moments later, they'd answer as if nothing were out of the ordinary.

When my children soon came to visit, Debbie and Luanne wondered how I'd react to them. When Lucas and Raechel came up to the bed, my face immediately lit up and I said, "Hi, Lucas. Hi, Raechel. It's good to see you. You both look so tall."

When Leo came closer to me, I reached over and patted him on the head, hesitating. "Hi, little guy," I said smiling.

Debbie and Luanne looked at each other. I hadn't remembered his name. Debbie picked up Leo and sat on the edge of the bed. "Isn't it good to see Dad awake, Leo," she said.

I reached over, grabbed Leo's hand, and laughed. "It's good to see you too, Leo."

As more of my family and various doctors came to visit that day, it became obvious that both my short-term and my long-term memories were impaired. The fact that I thought Lucas and Raechel looked tall coupled with my inability to recognize Leo seemed to suggest that my long-term memory was suffering from a gap of years. When Debbie started to talk about a lakeside cabin we had recently purchased and I didn't know what she was talking about, my sister immediately said, "Did she say your cabin? No, that's *our* cabin she's talking about." Everyone in the room laughed. I looked around and laughed along with the others. The strained look on my face showed that I really had no idea why I was laughing.

At one point that day, a neurologist came into the room to conduct some tests on me. He asked me my name and I replied without hesitation. He asked me how old I was. I looked around the room, at the expectant faces of my family waiting for my answer, finally at the hospital bracelet on my wrist. I twirled it around as if hoping to find the answer written somewhere on the bracelet, then said, "Twenty-nine?"

"Yes," said Luanne. "That makes me 27 then." Everyone laughed. So did I.

"What season is it?" the neurologist asked.

I hesitated, looked around the room, then out the window at the snow that was still piled on the window ledge. "Summer?"

I laughed.

No one else did.

Do memories have a purpose?

Memory can trap us. When we remember a certain event from the past, our present inevitably colours our memory. Paul Simon once sang about the Kodachrome colouring of the memories of his past loves — how everything looked worse in the stark reality of black and white.

My memories were not only un-Kodachromed, they were often unretrieved. I was trapped in a time warp of a present that had become limited to a framework of mere minutes at times. The past was hazy. The future was unfathomable. I had only the now.

Living in the now has long been touted as the goal for fulfill-ment in life, as the best way to live in order to achieve understand-ing. Ironically, I was restricted to the now by my faulty mem-ory. I could go no further. I wasn't just living in the now; I was languishing.

9

FIVE-MINUTE MEMORY

"Who was that?" I asked.

"That was the neurologist," Debbie calmly explained. "He came to see you earlier today."

"Oh, right."

"Why are we in the hospital?" I asked after a few seconds.

"You're in the hospital, Greg. I'm here visiting you."

"Oh, right."

How many times can I ask the same question?

Several people, including a steady stream of doctors and nurses, walked into my room the day I fully emerged from my coma. I greeted each visitor warmly and chatted amiably with them all. After each person left the room, I would turn to Debbie, who rarely left the chair at my side, and ask, "Who was that?"

She would calmly explain even though the nurse or doctor had invariably been in my room earlier that day or even moments before. After listening to Debbie's explanation, I would smile and say, "Oh, right."

The pattern continued throughout the day. I seemed to be unable to retain any memory for more than five minutes. All of my family members kept up a constant, unwavering dialogue with me.

"Why are we in the hospital?"

"You're in the hospital, Greg. We're here visiting you."

"What happened to my hand?"

"You fell at the end of a race."

"When can we go home?"

"You have to stay for awhile."

"Why are we in the hospital?"

Throughout those repeated conversations, I looked cheerful. Sometimes I would pause after a response, looking puzzled. Often, I would laugh as if I knew this seemed absurd. But then I'd ask the same question again.

How can short-term and long-term memories be so different?

Early in the afternoon, a young doctor carrying a clipboard walked in. I looked up from my bed, smiled broadly, and said, "Hi, Jason. What are you doing here?"

The doctor walked up to me, shook my hand, and said, "Hi, Mr. Marchand. I thought this was your chart."

I turned to Debbie. "This is Jason Wale. I taught him English in high school."

Debbie was shocked. She had been answering the same questions I posed to her over and over all day, and here I recognized a
former student without hesitation.

Jason talked about how much he had enjoyed my English
class, and I reminisced about watching him run cross-country
races the year the school team won the provincial championship.
It was the most sustained conversation I had had since I came
out of the coma. Jason explained that he had recently graduated
from medical school and was now doing his cardiac residency
working with Dr. Fretz, my cardiologist. He explained that he
just wanted to come in to see me and would be back shortly with
the cardiologist to explain what procedures they would be carrying out next.

Debbie was excited. So was the nurse who came into the room
soon after Jason left.

"You're lucky to have him working on your case," the nurse explained. "He's the star resident on this ward."

We continued to converse. I would doze off periodically while
nurses checked on me. My family tried to entertain each other
when I was asleep and entertain me whenever I was awake.

Later that afternoon, Dr. Fretz, followed by Jason, came in. I
glanced at Dr. Fretz, who had examined me twice that day, noticed
Jason behind him and said, "Hi, Jason. What are you doing here?"

Jason looked over at Debbie, puzzled.

"Sorry, Jason. His memory's a little off." She turned to me.
"Jason was in earlier this afternoon. Don't you remember?"

"Oh, right," I said. And laughed.

Dr. Fretz and Jason explained that the next test I would

undergo was a coronary angiogram. An angiogram is an x-ray that is used to view the coronary arteries on the surface of the heart. They explained how a cardiac surgeon would insert a catheter into a blood vessel in my groin and guide it up to my heart. He would then inject a dye through the catheter that would run to the coronary arteries and allow the x-rays to view them. The resulting pictures would reveal any possible abnormalities such as blockages or aneurisms in my coronary arteries. Because angiograms were performed at the Royal Jubilee Hospital only, they had arranged for an ambulance transfer the next morning. They explained that the angiogram would take place the next afternoon so advised me to get some sleep. Not needing any encouragement, I closed my eyes.

Author William Gibson wrote, "Time moves in one direction, memory in another." My memory had not yet decided on a direction to move. To a certain extent, my memories were stuck in the present. Yet my recollections were able to span decades. I was trying to remember events occurring around me. Largely, I was unsuccessful. Yet I was remembering a past that brought me little understanding of the present.

My memories were scattered. They were shaped by the details of my collapse that my family and doctors told me about, but were beginning to be influenced by the creeping truths I was gradually becoming aware of. My laughing responses to questions about my memory hid the gaps I was experiencing. Or at least I was trying to make them hide those gaps.

My memories were not just moving in a different direction

from time, but they were drifting uncontrollably. I wasn't the captain of my ship of memories. I was a passenger staring agog as I drifted. I was simply there for the ride not knowing the destination, not recognizing any of the landmarks along the way.

10

CORONARY ARTERY DISEASE

"Greg, you've got to keep still." Debbie held down my chest as she knelt on the gurney. At the foot of the bed, Luanne held my leg.

"You've got to keep this sandbag on your leg so it won't move," Luanne said as she struggled to keep me still.

"Why do I need a sandbag?" I asked, laughing, trying to stand up, and wondering why I felt so cold.

I shivered, continuing to wiggle around and laugh. I had no idea why they were being so serious. Why couldn't they just let me get up and let me move my leg?

"This is serious," Debbie said. Despite her words, she couldn't help but laugh herself.

Finally Debbie managed to get my attention. "Greg," she said using her best, stern, schoolteacher voice, "you've just had an angiogram. The doctor said that you have to stay still to prevent swelling in your leg. You've got to stop moving."

"But I'm cold."

Are angiograms dangerous?

Having been transported to the Royal Jubilee Hospital in an ambulance, I was blissfully unaware of the potential risks in undergoing an angiogram. The procedure itself can cause a heart attack; sometimes patients will have to undergo immediate, emergency bypass surgery; and as with all invasive procedures, patients can die. But I was still having trouble remembering why I was even in the hospital.

After being wheeled from my new room to a surgical procedure room on another floor, I had been given a simple, local anesthetic before a catheter was inserted into a blood vessel in my upper thigh. My first memory of the procedure, though, was feeling as if I had just come out of a general anesthetic. I was lying on a gurney in a hallway just outside the room where the procedure had been performed. Debbie and Luanne were on either side of the bed. In fact, Debbie was on top of the bed. My right leg seemed crushed under some weight I couldn't see. I was freezing. My body shook from the cold and I thrashed about trying to get the weight off my leg, trying to warm up. Ridiculously, I was laughing. Debbie and Luanne were laughing as well. But they were laughing out of frustration as they struggled to control me.

A nurse, noticing the predicament my wife and sister were in, came over and asked if they wanted a warm blanket for me. Debbie nodded gratefully. The blanket helped. It felt as though it had just come out of a hot dryer. I relaxed immediately. I still had no idea why I had to lie so still, but at least I wasn't shivering.

Debbie and Luanne continued to hold me steady, though,

fearing I would start to kick again at any minute. Debbie was still almost kneeling on my chest and Luanne clinging to my leg when Dr. Ofiesh, the cardiac surgeon, appeared. We hadn't moved from the hallway as we waited for an attendant to wheel me back to my room.

"I thought you would want to know right away," Dr. Ofiesh said. "I think we've found the problem."

My case had been a puzzle to everyone involved in it since I had arrived in the hospital. What would cause an otherwise healthy and fit 40-year-old to collapse while running a race, an activity that had become commonplace for him? With no history of heart disease or hypertension, no lifestyle activities that could be classified as risky, why would he suddenly go into cardiac arrest? Was it congenital, something he was born with? Was it an electrical imbalance in his heart? Or was it just simply unexplained sudden death? Dr. Ofiesh thought he had the answer.

"The angiogram shows Greg has coronary artery disease with severe blockages in at least two coronary arteries."

"What?" Debbie said, still trying to hold me down. "How could he have that?"

Again, I started to shift about like an unruly child not understanding that they were talking about me, about my heart.

"That's a good question. Usually, blockages like this are found in much older men who've made poor lifestyle choices: people who smoke or get little exercise. Why Greg would have coronary artery disease isn't clear. The blockages could have resulted from some childhood illness or genetic predisposition."

I had stopped fidgeting and was listening. Freed from

monitoring my leg, Luanne asked, "So he could have been living with this for years?"

"Yes. In fact the angiogram shows that his body has developed a complex set of collateral arteries that have been feeding blood to his heart for some time."

"What does that mean?" asked Debbie.

"We all have collateral arteries on the surface of the heart which are smaller than the coronary arteries. Greg's are more developed than any I've seen. They may be a result of his running over the years. But they've formed what are essentially natural bypasses around the blockages. They've probably kept him alive for years."

Debbie and Luanne were astounded. I lay listening but inattentive.

"What happens next?"

"Well, I would recommend bypass surgery."

Do they really stop your heart during bypass surgery?

Coronary Artery Bypass Graft Surgery (CABG, or "cabbage" as it is colloquially known) was first pioneered in the late 1960s. Today, over 500,000 bypass surgeries are performed every year in Canada and the United States. A bypass on a highway is usually built to speed up traffic. A typical road bypass allows cars to avoid traffic lights and inevitable congestion. Heart bypass surgery does the same thing. If an artery is blocked for any reason, blood flow lessens, reducing the amount of oxygen-rich blood delivered to the heart just as traffic congestion on the highway slows down cars moving through an intersection.

Bypassing a blockage can eliminate the decrease in blood flow to maximize the oxygen moving to the heart. Of course it's invasive surgery. The patient is first given a general anesthetic and then the heart surgeon cuts the patient's sternum bone down the middle and opens his chest. The patient is then placed on a heart and lung bypass machine so that the blood flow can be redirected and the heart stopped to allow the surgeon to work on it while it's not beating. The surgeon will have already harvested veins from the patient's leg or forearm or will redirect a mammary artery above the heart to use in the bypass. The harvested vein or artery is grafted on to the aorta above the blockage and then sewn below the blockage to allow blood to flow around it. Taking a vein or artery from one part of a patient's body and attaching it to an artery before and after a blockage is a serious bit of sewing. Sometimes the arteries or veins used are thinner that a strand of hair. Imagine trying to sew a hair onto another piece of hair. That's what a surgeon has to do with a bypass graft. Once he's finished, the heart is restarted, the patient taken off the bypass machine, his sternum stapled together, and his chest sutured.

Dr. Ofiesh didn't explain the whole procedure to us then. I wouldn't have been able to remember what he said anyway. But Debbie and Luanne, and the rest of my family, now had something tangible to prepare for.

I signed a form giving Dr. Ofiesh permission to perform his sleight of hand on me. But I had no idea what I was signing. I knew nothing of the potential risks associated with bypass surgery. I didn't know that by allowing a heart and lung machine to take the place of my newly stopped heart, I was risking further brain damage. I didn't know that both the chest and leg incisions were prone to infection following surgery. I didn't know that the staples holding my chest together would remain in my body, that I would be able to feel them through my skin, and that they would later set off alarms when I went through airport security.

I was oblivious to any possible concerns associated with CABG. I was blissfully oblivious.

11

DRIFTING WITH MORPHINE

"He'll be fine," my mother reassured Debbie. "You go home and have some time for yourself. Enjoy your lunch."

Two days before my scheduled heart surgery, my parents convinced Debbie to go home for a break while they stayed with me. Reluctantly she had agreed to go. It felt nice visiting my parents on my own.

"Let's go for a walk," I suggested after we'd talked for a short while.

"Oh, Greg, do you think you can?" my mom asked, her face showing her concern.

"Sure. I feel good today. I'd enjoy a walk."

I swung my legs across the bed and down towards the floor. The cold, hospital linoleum startled me and I searched for my slippers. My dad helped me find them while my mom held up my hospital gown.

"I don't need that," I said to her. "I have these nice pajamas you bought me."

The day after my parents arrived, my mom had asked Debbie if she thought she could bring some pajamas from home so that I wouldn't have to expose my backside in one of the notorious hospital gowns.

"Well, he doesn't really have any," Debbie had said. And then added quickly noting my mother's puzzled look, "He wears his boxers and t-shirt."

"Well, I'll get him some."

The plaid flannels I was now wearing were the first pair of pajamas she had bought me in over 20 years. I clung to the IV pole as I shuffled out the door, my parents on either side of me. It was a decidedly slow shuffle, but I was glad to be upright and proud that I could actually get around.

Why do I push myself even while I'm pushing an IV pole?

"Can you remember the last time the three of us had a stroll together?" I asked.

"Maybe when you were three," my dad said.

"Oh, Lou." This was my mom's usual response to a joke from my father that she didn't approve of.

We passed the nurses' station. Donna, who had become my most frequently helpful nurse and my favourite, was standing behind the counter writing on a chart. "Well, look at this," she said, "a parade."

I smiled. "Yeah, a parade in slow motion."

We shuffled by. I was still smiling by the time we reached the end of the hallway, but I was becoming visibly tired.

My mom noticed my weariness. "I think we'd better go back, Greg."

"No, I'm fine," I said, stubbornly proud.

"We've gone pretty far," said my dad. "Let's turn around here."

I agreed, realizing they both were right.

By the time we made it back to my room, I was perspiring and out of breath. My dad helped me back into bed, my mom not able to hide her emotions.

"We shouldn't have gone so far," she said. "Debbie will be so upset. Are you feeling okay?"

"Just a little tired," I said.

"What about your chest?"

"It's a little sore."

My mom didn't hesitate, but left the room to summon a nurse. It wasn't Donna who returned with her, but a much younger nurse. She had picked up my mom's concern and looked worried herself.

"How are you feeling?" she asked.

"A little sore."

"Where are you feeling sore?"

"Just a little in my chest."

"I'll get some nitro."

She was back in seconds, it seemed, with a small pill cup. The pill itself was tiny.

"Here, put this under your tongue," she said.

I opened my mouth and lifted my tongue for her to place

the pill under it. I could feel the effects almost immediately. My chest didn't hurt anymore, but I was struck by a blinding headache much more severe than the chest pain had been. My head throbbed and I couldn't keep my eyes open.

"Are you okay?" the young nurse asked.

"My head," I said. "It's pounding."

"That's a side effect of the nitro," she said, sounding knowledgeable but looking alarmed. "Is it bad?"

"Quite bad," I said, reluctant to admit to the pain.

"Do you need some morphine?"

"I don't think so."

"Maybe you should, Greg," said my mother, still worried that the walk had been too much for me.

"I'll get some," said the nurse.

If morphine is so bad for you, how come it feels so good?

I closed my eyes and tried to lie as still as I could. My dad reached over and began to massage my temples. The nurse returned with a syringe and a small bottle. She inserted the syringe into the bottle, extracted some fluid, and injected the contents of the syringe into the intake along the IV tube.

As with the nitro, it didn't take long before I began to feel the effects of the morphine. My breathing slowed and my heart seemed to beat more softly. I felt my whole body begin to sink slowly into the bed.

I heard the nurse asking me a question. It was something

about my head. I tried to concentrate on my head, the pain that had been there. I couldn't think. I began to tell her that I was feeling confused, but as I looked up, she was injecting something into my IV drip again.

The second dose of morphine hit me like a slow motion ocean wave. It washed over me gently, pushing me deeper into the softness of my bed. I felt as though I was drifting away from the room. I felt this strange battle within myself of relaxed euphoria and fear of losing control. The euphoria was beginning to win as I allowed myself to drift with the morphine.

From my haze, I became aware of Debbie walking into the room. I knew she would feel guilty for having left me. I knew my parents would feel responsible having taken me for a walk. I knew I would have to say something to them before I drifted away. I began to fight the euphoria again. I tried to assure them that I was okay, but I seemed to take several hazy minutes to even begin to speak. I tried to reach out from the morphine to tell Debbie that it wasn't my heart, but the narcotic that was causing me to act like this. I moved my arms, my hands beckoning, gesturing slowly, grandly. From the depths of my haze, I watched the movement of my hands. The slow, deliberate gestures reminded me of something. Of someone. Father Leo.

In 1990, Father Leo had died of liver cancer. At our wedding in 1980, he looked slightly jaundiced from a recent bout of hepatitis, which was probably the eventual cause of his cancer. He hated looking at our wedding photos because he thought he appeared yellow in them.

As he was in the hospital dying that summer, several of his friends set up a rotating schedule so that we could stay in his room overnight to keep him company. I stayed a few times. I remember reading to him, talking about our friendship while I was in university, and wishing that we had seen more of each other in the intervening years. Full-time teaching and children had begun to dominate my time.

I also remember watching Leo sleep. Brought on by doses of morphine, his sleep was fitful. He would awaken frequently and, even when he did sleep, his arms moved constantly. It was almost as if he were painting in the air or blessing a larger gathering. His hands moved gracefully, almost dancing. I cried for the beauty, the poetry of that movement.

My eyes had filled with tears as I struggled to say something to Debbie and my parents. Finally, feeling as if I were calling from the end of a long tunnel, I said, "I'm fine. Don't worry." I tried to smile, but Debbie looked worried.

"Are you sure you're okay?" Through her own tears, she asked, "Why are you crying?"

"I was thinking of Father Leo."

That evening, my mother talked to my three sisters about her afternoon at the hospital. She asked them to pray to Father Leo to watch over me.

How long does it take
for children to grow into their names?

When each of our children was born, we were very careful to try to choose names that were both singular and linked to our family histories. Lucas is a form of my father's name, Lucien. I actually had a dream that we should call him Lucas, not realizing the link to my dad. His middle names are James, my maternal grandfather's name, and Thornton, Debbie's maiden name. The spelling of Raechel's name is meant to emphasize the surname of Debbie's grandmother: Rae. Her middle names are Patricia, my mother, and Lorette, my paternal grandmother. We chose both names before Lucas was born, not knowing whether he was a boy or a girl.

We knew Leo's gender before he was born, however, so didn't have to think of two sets of names. I remember asking Debbie one night if she would mind if we called our third child Leo. She agreed immediately. She suggested Gregory as one middle name, and I suggested Thornton as the other. Lucas and Raechel loved the fact that they could speak to the growing bulge in Debbie's belly using his name. And when they came to visit their new brother in the hospital an hour after he was born, they had convinced Luanne and Keith, who drove them there, to pick up a stuffed lion as a gift for their new Leo. It wasn't the only stuffed lion he would receive, but it's still his favourite.

Leo's never been much of a ferocious lion by nature, though. Debbie told me a story about an early visit of his to see me in the hospital that suggests his nature is more akin to Father Leo's in some ways. Debbie had wanted him to have some time with me without his siblings present, to help jog my memory of him a little and to give him the time to begin relating to me again.

When they arrived, I opened the drawer beside my bed to offer him something to eat from the many gifts I'd received. I picked out some candy.

"Would you like a Lifesaver, Leo?" I asked, passing him the roll.

Leo slowly took the roll from me, and thoughtfully began to peel back the paper to expose the familiar centre hole of the candy. Instead of quickly taking a piece for himself, he handed the first one to me saying, "Here, Dad. You have a lifesaver. Then you won't die."

He handed the second one to Debbie. "You have one too, Mom." Not until he had watched us eat ours, tears welling in our eyes, did he take one for himself.

12

FATHER LEO

"Where are we?"

"In the hospital."

"Why are we in the hospital?"

"You're in the hospital, Greg. You fell at the end of a race."

The night after the morphine episode, Luanne stayed in my room with me answering the same questions repeatedly. She and Debbie had been alternating nights sleeping on a cot in my room. They feared I would wake up in the night, not know where I was, try to get out of bed, and pull the IV tube out of my arm or the heart monitor leads off my chest. I was still struggling with memory retention and would have to be reminded that I was in the hospital, especially when I awoke from a nap or a night's sleep.

Luanne slept little that night. I kept stirring or calling out. With every movement I made, she would wake up. Finally at about 4:00 a.m., I woke up completely. Luanne was awakened as well and reluctantly turned on the light. I began to ask the familiar questions.

"Where are we?"

"In the hospital."

"Why are we in the hospital?"

"You're in the hospital, Greg. You fell at the end of a race."

We cycled through those two questions and responses about 30 times. There were pauses in between. I'd remember something else from the past that we would talk about. But for almost two hours, I would invariably look around the room, get a puzzled look on my face, and ask Luanne, "Where are we?"

Luanne is an elementary school teacher and has infinite patience when patience is required. But she was drawing on all her classroom skills responding to my repetitions that night. Finally, when the cycle had come back to my "Where are we?" question, I unexpectedly said, "So I fell at the end of a race?"

When can the brain begin to heal on its own?

Luanne sighed gratefully. From that point on, our conversation changed. It became obvious to her that something was different. I didn't ask where we were. I responded to her questions. And I initiated conversation. Not only were my questions changing, but also it was the middle of the night, I wasn't tired, and I kept asking new questions. Luanne couldn't help but feel that I had turned a corner in my cognitive healing.

At one point, I asked a question that surprised my sister. Luanne and her husband Keith had been married for seven years. Keith had two grown daughters from another marriage, but Luanne had no children of her own. She and Keith had tried, but an operation to remove a uterine cyst she had when she was a teenager left Luanne with a remote chance of being able to conceive. Family means a great deal to Luanne. We're both very close to our two younger sisters who each have two daughters. And my children all adore Luanne.

Luanne and I had never really talked about her not having children. I knew it was a sensitive topic. But one of the consequences of the brain damage I had suffered that I wasn't cognizant of until much later, was the fact that I was more in touch with the emotions of others and the intangibles of life than I was with everyday realities. I was mere days removed from a brush with death and I was closer to that realm than I was to life around me. That night I broached the sensitive topic.

"How do you feel about not having children?"

The bluntness of my question startled Luanne. She had become accustomed to answering the same questions from me over and over again. This was a change.

She began slowly. "I've actually been thinking about that a lot lately. I'm not sure why. I guess it's from being here with you and seeing how much Mom and Dad have aged since the last time I saw them." She paused. I was still sitting quietly and listening.

"I guess I've started to realize that my role in the family may be different from everybody else's. Maybe I'm meant to be doing what I'm doing now. Helping you. And helping Mom and Dad when they get sick."

"But if you had children," I began.

"That's right," she continued. "If I had my own children, I

wouldn't be able to do that." She started to cry and I reached out to take her hand.

"It's funny. Realizing this has given me, I don't know, a real inner peace, a contentment that I've never felt before."

We were both in tears by that point. Although my memory was faulty, there was a part of my brain that understood the emotion behind Luanne's revelation, the pain she felt in letting go of a dream, and the healing power of the selfless attitude she was moving towards. We talked for hours that night, neither of us feeling the effects of a lack of sleep.

We didn't know it at the time, but Luanne was actually pregnant that night we spoke. She believes that she conceived on January 10th, the night before the race. Unfortunately, she miscarried two months later. She said to me later that she believes that, on some level, the life within her was used up to maintain mine.

We were both surprised, suddenly, to notice that the room had brightened. The sun had begun to rise. I excused myself and went into the bathroom to have a shower. Luanne later told me that I spent about 45 minutes in the bathroom. My memories of those 45 minutes are hazy. But they are the first tangible memories that I have of my hospital stay. I recall taking my time washing my hair and carefully toweling dry and shaving. I also spent time lost in thought.

Did I really see a ghost?

In the times of my life that I have conscientiously meditated, I've carried out that practice as my first activity of the day. Going slowly through the ritual of cleansing myself in the bathroom that morning, I was in a meditative state. In that state, I began to think of Father Leo. I could picture him clearly. He was a tall man, almost 6 feet 3 inches. And in the late 1970s when I first met him, he always wore heeled shoes that accentuated his height, making him an imposing figure. Everything about him seemed big. He had a full head of dark hair, a dark bushy beard that later became a dominant moustache, a strong but comforting voice, and large jewelry: always at least three enormous rings and usually a big wooden cross on a chain around his neck.

In the washroom that morning, after spending much of the night talking to my sister and having recalled him in a morphine daze the day before, I saw and, according to my sister, spoke to Father Leo. Luanne later told me that she heard me talking in the bathroom and knocked on the door on two different occasions to ask me if I was okay. In my image of Father Leo, he was wearing the unbleached cotton cassock he wore the day he married Debbie and me and he was bathed in a backlight that made his features unclear but his presence magnified. I remember feeling profoundly warmed by that presence and peacefully happy. His presence was so real to me that, as I walked out of the bathroom, I looked around the room expecting to see him there, waiting. Luanne was there instead.

I began to ask her about Father Leo, and then stopped. Not until that point had I remembered that he wasn't there, that he had died two hours after I had last visited him at the home of one of his parishioners having not wanted to die alone in the hospital, the very hospital that I was in at that moment.

This realization wasn't upsetting for me, however. Even though I understood he was dead, I continued to feel his presence. And this feeling seemed completely natural to me at that time. Yes, Father Leo was dead. Yes, I could sense that he was beside me. Yes, that understanding brought me comfort.

It's hard for me to clearly describe my experience of connecting with the spirit of Father Leo in the hospital. I believe that's exactly what it was though: a connecting with his spirit. I believe that some form of consciousness, some of the energy of those who have passed beyond this life continues to live on in this realm. I like to think of that as the spirit of the individual. The spirit of Father Leo was close to me when I was still closely connected to the other side, the realm that exists after death.

Becoming aware of his spirit was more than simply thinking of him. I felt his presence in the same way that we can often tell that someone is standing behind us even though we can't see that person. Twins have this same kind of connection with each other. Mothers and fathers have it with their young children. I had the connection with Father Leo in the hospital because I was still close to death myself; I was still loosely connected to this world. I had come back, aided by the CPR of the doctors on the roadside, by the prayers of the bystanders, by the entreaties of my family, and eventually by my own will.

The force of my will was definitely not strong at first, but eventually, I began to pull myself into this world. Father Leo was part of that pull. His reality in my world, his spiritual presence that I felt so strongly, coincided with my cognitive recovery. What I most admired about Father Leo in life was the melding of his keen intellect and spiritual understanding. As a chaplain in a university setting, he constantly lived that link. He was surrounded by colleagues and students in an intensely intellectual world, but was able to balance that cognitive side with his spiritual understanding. More importantly, he was able to articulate that balance to those who knew him, listened to him speak, or simply spent time with him. I attended Father Leo's masses, marveling at his sermons that weekly expressed his intellectual/spiritual balance, but I also played squash with him and attended several parties at his home.

So the pivotal presence of his spirit in my recovery was appropriate. The only way I would be able to bring myself back from the precipice of death was if I were able to find a material/spiritual balance in this world. Father Leo embodied that balance for me in life, and he presented it to me again in death.

The day I first felt his presence was the day my brain really began to heal. No longer did I ask the same question repeatedly. I still had lapses of memory and often struggled to find the correct word, the name of the nurse who had been on duty the night before, or even the birth date of one of my children. But from that day on, I noticed a change in my understanding, as did everyone around me. And those changes continued to occur regularly. They would come with literal flashes of insight. Almost as though a cartoon light bulb had illuminated in my head, I would suddenly become aware of something that had eluded me to that point. It wasn't always something specific like the title of a book or the date of a peace treaty. The flashes were moments where I realized that my brain had repaired, that a new pathway had formed, and that I was getting better.

Invariably, those first moments of insight were associated with a memory of Father Leo. Five or six times in the next year, I felt the synapses in my brain making those new connections. During that time, I was also acutely aware of Father Leo. I remember running into friends who had known him as well and I would begin saying to them, "I saw Father Leo the other day," truly feeling for a moment that I had seen him and that my friend would want to know that. But I always stopped myself, never knowing how I'd actually be able to explain those feelings. When the moments of memory flashes stopped, so did my sense of Father Leo's day-to-day presence.

13

TORTUOUS AND
NARROWED ARTERIES

From the report of Dr. Ofiesh, the heart surgeon:
"The findings of the coronary angiogram were surprising
in that they showed what I have interpreted as being a proximal
LAD aneurysm that has thrombosed and been calcified. I believe
this is a fairly chronic situation. The LAD distally has been supplied primarily using collaterals from the right coronary artery.
In addition, collaterals from the circumflex coronary artery fill a
large principal diagonal coronary artery. The circumflex coronary
artery itself appears to be normal, except that there is some slight
aneurysmal dilatation in its very proximal aspect. Otherwise the
vessel is entirely normal. On the right-hand side, that coronary
artery in its distal aspect appears entirely normal and is dominant,
but again proximally there is clear abnormality, with the vessel ap-
pearing to be tortuous and narrowed in the 60–70% range. Again,
I suspect there is an actual aneurysmal dilatation, and all we are
seeing is the course of the channel through the aneurysm.

"I have explained to the family that the indication for surgery in his case is that his only ischemic signs and symptoms appear to be sudden death. Under the circumstances, he should be a candidate for surgery on this admission. He clearly has abnormal coronary artery vessels where bypass would be required, involving at least two of the three major vessels. I think the ventricular fibrillation is clearly ischemic in origin and will be resolved with bypass."

Our hearts are essentially muscles that pump blood throughout our bodies all day, everyday, throughout our lives. The heart muscle contracts as it pumps then relaxes 100,000 times every day. At 40 years, 2 months and 20 days old at the time of my cardiac arrest, my heart had contracted and relaxed approximately 1.468 billion times when it suddenly stopped.

There are two sides to the heart, each being a separate pump, and each side has two chambers. The upper chambers, the atria, collect blood; while the lower chambers, the ventricles, pump blood. The right side of the heart receives blood coming from veins throughout the body and pumps it to the lungs. The oxygenated blood from the lungs returns to the left side of the heart, which pumps the blood, now full of oxygen, to the tissues and cells of the body.

All that pumping requires blood for the heart muscle itself; this blood comes via the coronary arteries, which come off the aorta, the main blood vessel. My left anterior descending (LAD) artery was completely blocked by an aneurysm that had calcified. An aneurysm is a weakening in the walls of a section of the artery causing it to enlarge or sag into a balloon shape. Aneurysms can burst a blood vessel when they expand too far. Calcification is the hardening of the artery walls around the aneurysm. Aneurysms of the LAD are found in only .1% of all angiograms – that is why Dr. Ofiesh was surprised. Blockage of the coronary arteries had deprived my heart of oxygen, causing my heart attack. Dr. Ofiesh proposed repairing (by bypassing) at least two of those arteries.

I was surprised again the next time I saw my former student, Jason Wale, when he came to see me the day after my angiogram. Although he had visited more than once since that first time I saw him and had asked Debbie and me several questions about my health history, I still looked shocked when he told me, once again, that he was a cardiology resident. My short-term memory was improving, but very slowly.

"I saw the results of your angiogram," he told us, "and I think I may have discovered a possible cause of your arterial blockages. It fits with something you told me yesterday."

With help from my mother, Debbie had told Jason about the last time I had been hospitalized. I was 15 and had traveled with my cousin and her young family from Calgary to Estevan, Saskatchewan, to attend her brother's wedding. He had asked me to be one of his groomsmen. I was looking forward to the weekend. My parents weren't coming and I was hoping to take full advantage of my freedom.

We left Calgary late Friday afternoon intending to drive late into the night in order to arrive early Saturday morning, the day of the wedding. From the driver's seat of their large Buick, Gary, my cousin's husband, kept assuring me that the weekend was going to be memorable.

"Just wait 'til you see the bride's cousin, your partner in the wedding party," he said. "She's a sweetie. We're going to get the two of you so drunk." He laughed and took a quick look into the backseat. "Not you two, though," he said to his young sons seated next to me in the back of the car.

"You just be careful, Gary," warned my cousin seated next to him. "You don't want Auntie Pat coming all the way to Estevan after you."

I tried to imagine my mother coming after Gary as I drifted in and out of sleep during the drive to Estevan. The normally eight-hour drive took less than seven with Gary at the wheel. By the time we arrived I had slept a little, but leaning awkwardly against the backseat door had left me with a stiff neck. A restless night on a foldout cot in another cousin's spare room didn't help. I woke with a pounding headache and a neck that was now swollen as well as stiff. After the wedding rehearsal, I asked Gary to stop at a drugstore to buy some aspirin. He suggested that I buy some 222s with codeine. "You won't have to drink much to get loaded with those," he said.

As it turned out, my throat was so sore that I could barely swallow. The 222s hadn't helped. I was sweaty and dizzy, and my head still pounded. In the wedding pictures taken that day, I'm smiling gamely. But my eyes are glassy; my neck is so swollen that it bulges over the collar of the ruffled, blue tuxedo shirt I'm wearing; and my head is bent awkwardly to the side.

I didn't last long at the reception. My "sweetie" wedding party partner avoided me all evening, not wanting to come close to someone looking more like Frankenstein's monster than a wedding date. I went back to my cousin's early and tried to sleep, my head pulsating painfully and my neck still cocked awkwardly to the right.

I awoke the next morning with a temperature of 39°C. My cousin called his dad who immediately came to pick me up and drove me to the hospital.

My neck and throat were so swollen that I still couldn't eat or drink, so the hospital's emergency personnel admitted me and started an intravenous drip. My temperature had spiked, my neck continued to swell, the whites of my eyes had turned completely red, and I had developed a rash on the upper half of my body. Even my tongue was bright red. The doctors in the Estevan hospital had never seen anything like this.

So my mother did end up coming all the way to Estevan. When my doctor phoned her in Calgary, telling her that he had no clear diagnosis for my symptoms, she flew out immediately. She spent a week there consulting with medical personnel, visiting with me in the hospital, and staying with family. By the end of the week, the doctors could think of only one thing. Since my white blood cell count was elevated, they feared leukemia.

My mother and I flew back to Calgary as soon as the doctors thought I was stable enough, my neck still grotesquely swollen. After an airline employee had wheeled me onto the plane and seated me, a concerned flight attendant looked at my neck and whispered to my mother, "Do you think it'll burst when we get airborne?"

It didn't burst, but when we arrived in Calgary and I was wheeled into the airport, the looks on the faces of my sisters and my father who were there to greet us, told me that I must have looked shocking. I spent three more weeks in the hospital in Calgary. My symptoms gradually subsided and tests ruled out cancer. The only viable diagnosis that doctors could come up with was quinsy, something I'd never heard of before. Friends who visited me in the hospital said a rumour had spread around the school that I had alcohol poisoning.

Does Kawasaki disease have anything to do with motorcycles?

Jason looked excited. "You told me yesterday about your hospital stay when you were a teenager. Well, the symptoms you had then could have been attributable to something called Kawasaki disease."

Jason went on to explain that Kawasaki disease was first identified in Japan in 1967. I was hospitalized in the fall of 1972. It usually affects young children, but its origin is unknown. Scientists suspect a virus causes it. It is diagnosed when patients exhibit five or more of its classic symptoms: a persistent high fever between 38 to 40°C; a rash on the trunk and groin; irritation and redness of the whites of the eyes; swollen lymph glands in the neck; abnormal inflammation and redness of the mouth, lips, throat and tongue; and an elevated white blood cell count. In about 20% of cases, the coronary arteries are affected and often form aneurysms or blood clots that can lead to a heart attack.

My mother was in the room while Jason explained about Kawasaki disease. She was shocked. "You had every one of those symptoms when you were in the hospital."

"But you said it usually affects young children," Debbie said. "Greg was 15 when this happened."

"Well, that's the interesting thing," said Jason. "I read a study of some cases of Kawasaki disease striking patients in late adolescence. When these patients reached their 30s and 40s, many of them suffered heart attacks and sudden death, most of them brought on by exercise. Almost all of the patients exhibited arterial aneurysms, blocked arteries, and extensive collateral artery development. That sounds like you."

It did sound like me. My hospitalization as a teenager had been almost forgotten in our family. Probably because we had wanted to forget about it. The unknown origin of my ailment frightened us, especially my mother who had to endure traveling to Estevan on her own thinking that she was retrieving her dying son. Now, 24 years later, she had flown to Victoria, thinking the same thing.

But Jason had presented information that gave us an answer. He explained that coronary artery abnormalities associated with Kawasaki disease could be avoided by introducing intravenous gamma globulin early in the illness. Had I received that treatment in Estevan when I was 15, I probably wouldn't have suffered a cardiac arrest in Saanichton when I was 40. But how many doctors in Estevan, Saskatchewan, in 1972, had even heard about Kawasaki disease, something discovered only five years earlier on the other side of the world? And if someone had heard of it, I'm sure the

coronary artery abnormalities associated with it hadn't been ob-
served often enough by 1972 to even draw preventative conclu-
sions. If I had contracted a virus that developed into Kawasaki
disease when I was 15, I would never know. Nonetheless, I was
about to undergo open heart surgery to correct a highly unusual
aneurysm blocking one artery and a second vessel Dr. Ofiesh described as "tortuous and narrowed" that may have been damaged
by the disease.

14

IT DOESN'T SEEM RIGHT

"It doesn't seem right that you have to go through this," said the nurse as he pulled a razor across the hairs on my chest.

"Ouch," I said after he'd tugged at one stubborn section. "You're right, it doesn't seem right that I have to have my chest shaved."

"No, I don't mean that. I mean your heart surgery tomorrow. That's why I'm in here with my razor. I have three children at home too. They need me. And your kids need you too, so you need to get well so you can get back to them."

"Well, I'm planning to." I'd almost forgotten about the surgery. "It also doesn't seem right that the only male nurse on this floor is shaving me with all those good-looking women nurses out there."

"Well you're certainly feeling perky today, aren't you? What would your wife say about that?"

"She'd just laugh. Take a look at me. I'm quite a sight with all these chunks of hair out of my chest."

"What? You don't think I'm a good barber? Just wait till we get lower."

"What do you mean?"

"I have to shave that hair as well. That's why the women are out there and not in here."

"That's too bad."

"It doesn't seem right, does it?"

At what point does trying hard become trying TOO hard?

I didn't realize it at the time, but as I waited for my bypass operation, I was trying too hard. I tried too hard to understand. I tried too hard to remember. I tried too hard to think. Sometimes I would be able to relax and let life advance around me. But as I was able to remember more, the harder life seemed to be for me. Most of the time, my mind was still lost in the haze of forgotten memories. I was learning to cover myself well, though. When someone would tell me something and I'd react with a blank stare, that person would say, "You remember that, don't you?"

My response was always a laugh. "Of course. That's right," I'd say. And laugh.

Once I responded differently to my mother. I had just been transferred by ambulance to the Royal Jubilee Hospital, and she was in my new room alone with me. We were talking about her family and she mentioned her brother. My brain, working hard to keep up with her, suddenly presented me with the memory that he had been sick. "How is Uncle Phil?" I asked.

"Oh, Greg. Don't you remember? He died."

I was overcome. Like a bubble gently surfacing on a still

pond, the memory of my uncle's recent death from cancer slowly rose to my consciousness. I started to weep. "I had forgotten," I whispered.

My mom immediately tried to comfort me. "I'm sorry, Greg. I shouldn't have said anything." My emotions were raw and always close to the surface in those early days in the hospital. When I saw my parents standing at my bedside after they had flown immediately from Calgary, I broke into uncontrolled sobs. At some level, I must have realized that they had come to be with me, fearing that I wouldn't survive. Their presence was a sign that I was hovering, that death was near.

After she had calmed me down, my mother left my room to join my family in the waiting room. My two younger sisters, Colette and Allison, had just arrived from Calgary, having flown in to be with the rest of my family awaiting my operation.

Colette is six years younger than I am and definitely the most easy-going member of our family. I love, and envy, her relaxed attitude towards life. The only one of us siblings with a French given name, she has the same *joie de vivre* as our father whose own father was born in France. Her relaxed attitude extends to all aspects of her life from her creative culinary pursuits to her house cleaning. Colette has a plaque on her bedroom wall that reads, "I've never heard a famous person say, 'I owe it all to my mother's clean house.'"

Allison is my youngest sister and was only nine years old when I left home. For many years, I thought of her as I remembered her when I moved out: a cute blonde with slightly bucked teeth, a freckle-splattered nose, and brightly innocent eyes. We both remember a turning point in our relationship, though, when the two of us had coffee together on our own without children or other family members and were able to truly communicate with each other on an adult level. Since then, we'd had many adult conversations, and I'd come to appreciate her spiritual view of life and her contagious sense of humour.

After coming out of my hospital room, my mother told them about my reaction to remembering my uncle's death. Still upset with herself that she had revealed the truth to me, she advised the rest of them not to say anything that might upset me.

Allison, immediately said, "Well, for goodness sake, don't anyone tell him about Sonny Bono." Everyone burst into laughter. The absurdity of my reacting emotionally to the recent death of Cher's former husband was the kind of humour that defined the character of my family. We loved to laugh. Even in cardiac wards.

15

I WISH THEY'D
BRING BREAKFAST

"I know you've been waiting a long time this morning," said Dr. Ofiesh as he entered my room. "But I'm sorry. You'll have to wait just a bit longer. I've been in surgery all night and need some sleep before I can operate on you."

It was late in the morning, the day of my bypass surgery, and I had been fasting since dinner the night before. Debbie and I had been waiting through the delays together and she had not eaten either in support of me.

"Please, get as much sleep as you need," I said smiling and ignoring my growling stomach. "I want you to be at your best."

Why do they always give you popsicles in the hospital?

Debbie and I reluctantly settled in for a longer wait and a longer fast. A nurse brought us a Popsicle, the only food I was allowed to eat. We shared it.

"You can have something else to eat," I said to Debbie.

"That's okay. I'm not hungry."

"I am."

We waited.

I could sense Debbie's fear. I wasn't sure what she was afraid of.

"How are you feeling?" Debbie asked.

"I'm fine. Just hungry. I wish they'd bring breakfast."

"You're not allowed to eat. Remember?

"How come?"

"The operation."

"Oh, right."

16

POST OP

"What's going on? Why can't I open my eyes?"
I kept trying to open them, but my eyelids felt as though someone were pushing on them from above my head. A dull pain in my chest wouldn't go away. Someone must be pushing on it too, I thought. I could hardly breathe. I tried my eyes again. This time they opened a little more, but the bright lights made them burn. I wanted to just lie still, forget about my chest or opening my eyes.

Debbie was calling my name. Her voice drifted in from a distance as if she were on the other side of a lake, the sound bouncing over the water like a cast stone skipping several times before it reached me.

If I could open my eyes, maybe I could see where she was. I tried again, blinking, my eyelids flopping under the weight of whatever it was pushing on them. Through the flickering I could see Debbie, the brightness of the room almost obscuring her face. I sucked in a breath of air and tried to speak.

"Where am I?" I asked, through shallow breaths.

"You're in the recovery room," she said. "The operation went fine. You're doing really well."

"The operation?"

"Your bypass surgery. Remember? The doctor had to do a triple bypass in the end, but he said that it was a complete success. Your heart's fine."

"My heart?" I reached up to my chest. It was covered in a thick bandage.

"You shouldn't touch it, Greg," Debbie said. "Don't worry. It's fine. The surgeon said that he'd never seen such twisted arteries, though."

"Oh. Is that good?"

"It wasn't good. But now you have bypasses going around them."

"That's good." I closed my eyes and drifted off.

Do children worry about their parents too?

As I drifted in and out of consciousness in the hospital, my family waited to hear about the results of the operation. Some were at our home; some still lingered in the hospital waiting room. Months later, I mentioned to Luanne how, during my hospital stay, I was very aware of how hard it was for my Dad to be there. I remember consciously striving to make him feel it was all right when he would have to leave. I didn't want him to feel guilty. Later, I began to ponder why he felt that way. Even that pondering bothered me since I saw it as a by-product of my replenishing brain. When it was tougher for me to think and remember, I wasn't concerned about such issues as why my dad felt the way he did. I just accepted without worrying.

As Luanne and I spoke, she told me a story about when Mom and Dad were staying at her house soon after their arrival in Victoria. Mom was in the kitchen helping Luanne clean up and Dad was in the living room reading the paper. Dad then came into the kitchen whistling. Mom turned to him saying, "How can you whistle at a time like this?" Dad didn't respond but sheepishly left the room. Twenty minutes later, Luanne looked out the window to the deck. Dad was there, leaning on the railing with rosary beads in his hand, praying. She said he had his rosary beads with him constantly.

Luanne also told me about the evening they were all at our house waiting to hear from Dr. Ofiesh about the results of the by-pass operation. Everyone was in the living room when the phone rang. Debbie, who had been waiting to return to the hospital, rushed to answer the call, returned with the good news, and burst into tears. Everyone else began to cry as well, releasing the emotions they had held in check for 11 days. Luanne said that Mom and Dad were sitting at opposite ends of the couch and when they heard the news, Mom slid across the couch and put her head against Dad's chest. For several minutes, they both sat there hugging and crying.

It pained me to hear that. Part of the issue for me was imagining my parents being so demonstrative. I supposed that my sisters and I must have longed for them to be that way since they rarely were. And, of course, part of my emotional response to the image of the two of them crying was knowing that my cardiac arrest and surgery had elicited their actions. It was hard for me to come to terms with the notion that I had affected all of them in such a way, that what had happened to me was responsible for perhaps the greatest pain that any of them had felt to that point.

17

CLUTCHING PILLOWS
INSTEAD OF FOOTBALLS

"My heart seems to be so loud now," I told Dr. Ofiesh when he came to visit me the day after he had operated on me. "I can hear it beating all the time. Is that because it's working better now?"

He laughed. "No, I don't think it's working better. Your arteries are circulating blood better, but your heart is pumping the same. If anything, it's working less strenuously than it was before the surgery. A lot of patients say they can hear their hearts more. I think you're just more aware of it."

Of course I was more aware of it. That's all I thought about. My heart had stopped twice: two weeks ago on a country roadside and two days ago in an operating room. I didn't want it to stop again any time soon.

When do we begin to watch sports more than play them?

After the births of our children, I would take Debbie for walks around the maternity ward in the hospital to help her regain her strength and prepare for the move home. We'd pass other mothers slowly moving down the hall as well. They called their painful, deliberate gait the episiotomy shuffle. After my heart surgery, Debbie led me on walks around the cardiac ward. My gait was just as deliberate as Debbie's had been. My own bypass shuffle included clutching to my chest a heart-shaped pillow. Every time I coughed, which was often, I'd pull the pillow tighter to my chest trying to alleviate the pain. It hurt. But I had to cough to make sure my lungs didn't fill with fluid. I felt as though I was holding my heart in place, preventing it from leaping through my stapled together sternum and sewn together chest.

That evening the ward seemed quieter than usual. Surprisingly, I had no visitors, and I hadn't noticed any other heart surgery patients passing by. I decided to go for a walk myself. Once in the hall, I heard the sound of cheers and the occasional groan coming from the common room at the end of the corridor. Clutching my pillow, I shuffled down.

The room was filled with patients, all of them male, most of them overweight. They were watching a football game. I suddenly realized it was Super Bowl Sunday. I wasn't a big NFL fan, but I was always aware of the date of the game that stopped time every winter throughout much of North America. I wanted to join in the conversation with a manly, "How about them Patriots?" But I had no idea who was playing. And I was too embarrassed to ask.

So I leaned against the wall, clutched my pillow, coughed occasionally, and tried to enjoy the game.

It didn't take me long to lose interest in watching football, however. What did interest me, was the makeup of the audience. Looking around the sea of balding heads, I realized that I was by far the youngest man there and I was at least 20 pounds lighter than anyone else. As I watched one of them grab a handful of potato chips from a bowl in the centre of the room, I began to think of the nature of heart disease. Every year, more than 500,000 North Americans die of heart attacks. Most of them are men. And many of them have unhealthy lifestyles. Cardiovascular disease is the leading cause of death in both men and women in North America. Twice as many people die from cardiovascular disease as die from all types of cancer. Yet we continue to lead sedentary lives, watching sports instead of participating in them, while our arteries clog.

The irony of my smug observations, as I stood leaning against the wall, was that we were all clutching pillows. We were all cringing in pain as we coughed. We were all conscious of the scars running down our chests and the shallow breaths we were sucking in. We were all heart patients. Our lives to this point might have been different, but we were now an unlikely group of comrades.

"Have a seat," a man next to me said in between coughs, indicating a chair next to him.

"Thanks," I said, and sat down to watch the rest of the game.

18

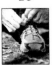

GOING HOME

"You think you're going home today, don't you?" Nurse Donna said to me.

"Do you think he'll let me?"

"I don't know. How long has it been since your operation? Four days?"

"Yeah, but look at me." I stood up and struck what I hoped was a manly pose of strength, but immediately tottered back onto the bed.

Donna laughed. "At that rate, you'll be in here another week." I knew she was teasing, but I felt dejected.

She smiled. "Don't worry. Let's take a look at your vitals before Dr. Ofiesh gets here."

After Donna checked my blood pressure and temperature, recording the results on my chart, she walked out, leaving me to prepare for the surgeon's visit.

Is it good to feel competitive about leaving the hospital?

I had awakened that morning cautiously optimistic, thinking about the possibility of being discharged from the hospital when my surgeon made his rounds later in the morning. It was a Friday, and I couldn't imagine Dr. Ofiesh making me stay in the hospital for the whole weekend. He had told me that four days would be the minimum stay in the hospital after bypass surgery. I was competitive enough to want my stay to meet that standard.

After breakfast, I quickly washed up and shaved. At least I tried to be quick. Speed for me was now a relative term. From the moment my head hit the gravel road at the end of the race, speed was nothing like it had been before. Washing, shaving, and dressing were all exhausting, and painfully slow acts. And the deliberate processing of my brain slowed my actions even more. Looking in my shaving kit in the bathroom, I'd find myself puzzling over the purpose of the tin of shaving cream or the necessity of the multi-coloured bristles on my toothbrush. When I was finally able to lather my face with shaving cream, I'd dig thorough the contents of my kit bag several times unable to locate the apparatus that I knew I'd need to complete the job of shaving. Even the shape of the razor was a puzzle to me.

When I finally finished in the bathroom, washed and clean-shaven, I sat on the edge of my bed and waited. Finally, I heard Dr. Ofiesh's familiar voice at the nursing station. I sat up as straight as I could when he entered my room with his usual commanding air.

I tried encouraging as much healthy-looking colour in my face as possible. He looked stern.

"So, how are you feeling?"

"Great."

"Are you sure?"

"Never better."

"Well, that's probably a bit of a stretch." He paused as he read my chart while I watched him with growing anxiety. Finally, he looked back at me and smiled. "But I don't see why we should keep you around here anymore. You can go home."

I wanted to jump up and hug him but thought better of it knowing that kind of energy expenditure wasn't a good idea. Instead, I held out my hand. "I can't thank you enough, Dr. Ofiesh."

He reached over and shook my hand. "You're welcome. Now it's your job to get stronger."

"That's exactly what I plan to do."

The moment he was out the door, I phoned Debbie. I tried to pack up the room before she arrived but had the energy to do little more than dress myself. Debbie and my mom soon arrived with a small suitcase for me and a basket of baked goods for the nurses. They helped me pack up the few clothes I had and the dozens of cards displayed around the room. My feelings were tinged with emotion as we said goodbye to the nurses. These women and men had cared for me and my family as if we were their own family. I liked them. And I felt as though they genuinely liked us as well. But I had no idea how I could begin to express my gratitude to them. All I could do was hug them to my bandaged chest as I choked back tears.

Is bypass surgery an efficient way to lose weight?

It was a crisp winter day, the sun shining as I shuffled out the front door of the hospital. I gratefully breathed in the fresh air. The last time I had been outside was three weeks before as I lay on a gravel road, not breathing in any fresh air at all. It was a short, five-block drive from the Royal Jubilee Hospital to our home, but I enjoyed sitting in the front passenger seat, looking out the window at the familiar streets, houses, and trees that appeared vibrantly new to me in the sunlight.

I carefully stepped out of the car when we arrived home, walked the few steps to the stairway at the front of our house, and then laboured up the five or six stairs. At the top, I stopped, out of breath, and sat on a wicker chair on our front porch. It was a glorious day, and I drank in the beauty, reveling in my liberty and life.

We have a photograph that Debbie took of me sitting on the porch that day. In the photo, I look happy but pale, my usual ruddy complexion hidden behind pasty grey skin. My always-unruly hair hasn't been cut or combed in weeks. It sticks up and out looking almost comically large and making my face look thinner than it should have. My face was indeed thinner. I weighed my usual 165 pounds the day of the race. When I was weighed on my discharge from the hospital, I was 20 pounds lighter.

Smiling for the camera, I was happy. I was happy to be home, happy to sit outside, happy to be breathing in this crisp, late January air. The sun brightens the background in the photo. I remember that sun. I remember sitting on the porch for several minutes until Debbie came out to get me. "It's cold out here, Greg. You'd better come in."

Why do we so easily forget to appreciate the beauty of a bird's nest?

It didn't feel cold to me. It felt clear and fresh and alive. I felt alive. I remember sitting on that porch often in those first few weeks of my recovery. I could watch people walking by on the street, leading their dogs or pushing their children in strollers. I could smell the damp freshness of the earth. I could listen to the birds perched in the stark, leafless branches of the overgrown Japanese plum tree in our front yard.

Another tree next to the house, a smoke bush that had grown past the bush stage and now snaked its way up to the second storey of the house, became a fascination for me. In it, a pair of small birds was painstakingly building a nest. I watched the construction for several weeks that spring until the bush began to grow leaves again covering the nest. They were tiny birds, bushtits I later found out. Their nest looked more like a grey tube sock made of mud, grass, and twigs. It was almost a foot long while the birds themselves were only a few inches tall. The nest grew in length daily as I watched it becoming for me the image of the rebirth of spring, the shelter for the new life that eventually emerged within it.

The central doctrine of Christianity, like the essence of spring, is the belief that death brings rebirth. It was January 27th, but the promise of spring was evident. Debbie had taken all the bulbs and flowering plants that I had received in the hospital and had planted them in a separate spot in our front garden. Some were still flowering, some were about to, and some had already passed the flowering stage. But they were all evidence of the cycle of death and rebirth that spring symbolizes.

In that spring-like fresh air, I was simply reveling in my freedom, drinking in the life that pumped through my grafted arteries. I thought of the symbolism of that moment. I embodied that central premise of Christianity. My death and rebirth were as evident as the daffodils in the garden Debbie had planted. The bulbs that had lain dormant over the winter were now alive with the promise of green stems and golden flowers. I was alive with the promise of survival.

When are the messages in dreams most important?

When I finally went in the house, I saw that Debbie had pulled out the sofa bed in our living room making it into a bedroom for us. She worried that I wouldn't be able to walk up the flight of stairs to our room my first day home and wanted me to be in a more central position in the house as well. But the bed was uncomfortable and I slept fitfully that first night. I had taken two Tylenol 3s and hallucinated most of the night.

One of those dream-like hallucinations centred on a dinner we were having at Debbie's sister's house. We were living in a house next to hers although we don't in reality. I had put the kids to bed after dinner and had then ventured downtown. It became dark and I began to worry about getting back to the kids. The downtown streets were full of late night revelers who unsettled me so much that I wanted to leave right away. But I couldn't find a way home. There were no buses or taxis. I began to walk, then run, but kept losing my way.

That same night, I dreamt about Debbie chastising me. She was upset that I was sick and that I wouldn't be able to do anything around the house to help her. I tried to convince her that I would do as much as I could but acknowledged that I was still very weak and wouldn't be able to do a great deal.

In a third dream, I was entering a swimming pool at a local recreation centre. As I walked in, I became aware of a number of young women looking at me. I felt flattered and proud. But then I suddenly realized that they weren't looking at me. They were looking at the scar on my chest.

19

MEN AND MORTALITY

"What are you looking at?"
"Stop looking at me."
"I said stop looking at me!"

I woke with a start, my heart pounding. I looked around, not sure where I was, the bed too soft. Then I remembered the sofa bed. And the dreams. I tried to calm down, tried to make my heart slow its pounding. Debbie stirred beside me. Was I speaking out loud? She could probably hear my heart, I thought. This couldn't be good for it. Slowly, I slid out of bed, trying not to wake Debbie, and made my way to the bathroom.

I turned on the bathroom light and looked in the mirror. Seeing my reflection, I felt gaunt. Most of the 20 pounds I'd lost in the hospital seemed to come from my legs, arms, and chest. I'd looked skinny before, but now I was a wisp of my former self.

From the perspective of a man, these last three weeks had been profound. Men don't contemplate their mortality much. For my 40th birthday, I had thought about parachuting from a plane. The thrill of falling through the air excited me. I didn't imagine the possibility of dying. But Debbie was upset about the prospect of my doing it: she thought about dying. Eventually understanding her perspective, I didn't go.

Men are typically lax about going to the doctor. We don't like standing naked in front of a practitioner while being prodded and poked. Visiting a doctor is an admission of frailty. And we don't like to feel frail.

My reflection continued to stare back at me. My arms looked wimpy and my gut stuck out. Even more disconcerting was the long scar running down my chest from the base of my neck to my navel. Everything had changed too much, and I hated being faced with such an altered state. I shuffled out of the bathroom and went back to the sofa bed.

Can we ever be sure of the exact cause of any illness?

In the weeks and months following my cardiac arrest, I had ample time to think, to read, and to wander the house. When I looked at old photographs of myself scattered about our home – family photos in calendars and on tabletops – I couldn't help wondering about the state of my heart when the photo was taken. When did my arteries start blocking up? Had they started clogging when that picture of my sisters and me was taken when I was eight? When were the blockages most dangerous? In that photo of me skiing last year? How long had I been a walking time bomb? In all of these pictures?

I wanted to be able to look back and see the events in my life that slowly and over time led to the blockages. A piece of cheese-cake here. Stifling a painful memory there. An angry, frustrated outburst at someone. Did events like those have the most profound effect on my coronary artery disease? Or had it always been there? Did it start with a virus in my childhood?

My cardiologist said that my lifestyle and age put me in the smallest imaginable percentile for developing this disease. I beat the odds contracting it. Yet I beat the odds surviving it as well. Very few live through a cardiac arrest on the street the way I had. Most who survive are already in the hospital and have the advantages of medical personnel and technology at their immediate disposal. That's why the intervention of those doctors was so vital for me at the race. I couldn't have collapsed at a better place outside a hospital.

I realized that I would never truly know all the causes. That's why the cardiologist who treated me in the hospital was so adamant about keeping me on a cholesterol-lowering drug. Cholesterol does cause blockages in the arteries so my best defence against those was keeping my cholesterol low. I still thought I could control my cholesterol levels through diet and lifestyle. Taking the drug made me uneasy, so I felt I needed the chance to try dealing with my body without daily doses of a harsh medication. Even its makers admitted to not understanding how it worked.

Wanting to try alternative forms of healing, I met with acupuncturist Dr. Michael Greenwood about a month after my bypass surgery. When I brought up the subject of medication, he asked me why I didn't just stop taking it. Thinking about his question for a moment, I acknowledged that I was scared. I feared that stopping it would increase my cholesterol levels. He said that maybe his acupuncture treatments would allow me to overcome that fear enough to let me give it up.

Having read a book he'd written about alternative medicine and healing, I was beginning to understand his thinking. He sees illness as having underlying causes that aren't always the most obvious. My heart problems might have had their genesis in something completely removed from cholesterol. The reason I would want to continue racing, despite the fact that it seemed to be the cause of my cardiac arrest, might have held the key to that underlying cause. Was I too driven to succeed for my own good? My running was such a paradox. The collateral arteries that formed around the blockages in my arteries, largely because of the fitness level I'd attained by running, kept me alive for years. Yet pushing my body to its physical limits while running finally caught up to me on that gravel road in Saanichton.

Running can be a reflective endeavour. Often my runs became almost meditative for me. At times, I think I'd used them to take me beyond the temporal world around me. Periodically, I thought myself too immersed in the world. Early on in my recovery, I definitely wasn't centred on worldly concerns. Sometimes I longed to be in that position again. "The world is too much with us," Wordsworth wrote. "Getting and spending we lay waste our powers." Whatever powers I may have had, I feared laying waste to them, not just by the getting and spending, but by all the everyday concerns of the world. I left my meeting with Dr. Greenwood seriously considering visiting him again for a treatment.

*Was I ready to come back to
the reality of everyday life?*

One day shortly after my return home after the bypass surgery,
Debbie and I went to a nearby shopping mall together. I stopped
to deposit a cheque at the bank just outside the entrance while
she walked ahead into the mall. After depositing the cheque, I
continued into the mall. All around me, shoppers jostled with
each other as they hurried from store to store. They seemed to
be everywhere, and their pace felt far too frenetic for me. I looked
through the crowd of shoppers for Debbie. She was nowhere in
sight.

A wave of fear began to surge through me. I wasn't sure what
to do. I couldn't see Debbie anywhere and I felt even more panicked as I became swept into the crowd of shoppers while I looked
for her. People surrounded me and they were moving quickly, like
a pack of runners at the beginning of a race. I took a deep breath
and tried to reassure myself. "It's just a mall," I told myself. "These
are shoppers just going about a normal activity. Debbie's probably
in the shoe store straight ahead."

It took me a few anxious moments, but I was able to calm
myself. I walked through the crowd of shoppers and soon found
Debbie in the very store I'd thought she was in. But that sudden
onset of panic scared me. It scared me because I knew I could have
easily slipped further into that panicked state and gone beyond it.
I knew that I could have lost myself in the fear. Although the pan-
icky feeling didn't last long, I realized how close to the edge I still
was. And oddly, that edge was a little appealing.

When people visited with me in the hospital or just after I had returned home, I had few expectations for myself and most of my visitors expected little from me as well. I could drift off in my thoughts; I could even drift off to sleep. I was like the protagonist in Margaret Atwood's novel *The Edible Woman* who, in the middle of a small gathering, quietly slips between a bed she's sitting on and the wall until she's under the bed and out of sight. She feels comfortable and safe there. But then she has to reappear, rise from beneath the bed to encounter the others in the room. Of course, they've all seen her slide down and are staring dumbfounded when she reappears. She was expected to act somewhat normally.

I was expected to act that way as well. I'd slid down beneath the bed and now had re-emerged myself. But I wasn't sure how ready I was to be back. Before my mind began to clear and my memory started to return, I would smile or laugh at questions posed to me. "What's your middle name, Greg?" I'd laugh. "What city were you born in?" I'd look around me. "Not here, I hope." I'd laugh. Everyone else would laugh as well. But I must have been worried. I always kept trying. I wanted to answer the questions correctly. I just wasn't able to.

A few months after my surgery, I was answering most of the questions correctly. I was thrilled with the progress I'd made. But I couldn't help remembering how much easier it was when I simply had to laugh.

With that simplicity of vision and understanding came an intuitive knowledge that I felt was slipping. I dreamt of events that would occur the next day. I seemed to understand the emotions behind a comment made to me. I was relying on intuition instead of knowledge. My brain couldn't remember, but my heart could.

I felt afraid of losing that connection to my heart. I still wanted to intuit. I'd been fighting to regain knowledge, but I wondered what I'd lost as a result of the gains I'd made.

Where do we find our own truths?

Walking home from the library one spring afternoon, I felt happy and contented. The sun was warm and my brisk pace refreshed me. Acknowledging that sense of inner peace, I felt I had come to an important realization about myself and about the direction I was heading. I knew I had no need to do anything but what I was doing then. I could write, exercise, look after Leo, who was the only one home with me now that everyone else had gone back to school, and keep my mind clear and my heart healing. There was nothing compelling me to do anything but remain healthy. The less I filled my head and days with the pre-January 11th clutter in my life, the more room I had for what was truly meaningful. I still felt driven, but I was learning to let go, to simply trust.

I'd interviewed and published profiles of three different people in the months directly after my cardiac arrest who'd told me that the successes they'd had in their lives were not truly their own accomplishments. They all believed a Spirit much greater than they controlled their lives. For the Roman Catholic Bishop Remi De Roo and university chaplain Kate Fagan, that Spirit was their Christian God. For sculptor Maarten Schaddellee, the Spirit was in the whales he watched, the stone he used to sculpt those whales, and the home next to the ocean in which he lived and worked.

Interviewing them was a lesson for me. They were all truthful in their comments. They all walked the talk they preached. I had to do the same. But I had to do so from within my own truth.

A few days after my interview with Maarten, I received a card from his wife Nadina who had been as much a part of the interview as her husband. In her card she wrote that during our visit, I had "looked transparent" and "between the worlds." She continued, "Your courage will come from standing in the centre of a place no one can see, knowing what no one can verify, and dancing to a tune no one else can hear."

I needed simply to let go and dance in order to find that courage.

20

LIKE A THIEF
IN THE NIGHT

"Do you remember this?" I asked Debbie as I passed her a handmade card.

We were sitting on the couch reading after the kids had gone to bed. She was reading a novel and I was leafing through some of the cards and letters I'd received while I was in the hospital.

"Of course I remember," she said. "Leo drew the pictures while he was waiting in the hospital one day. Then he dictated the captions for me to write under them."

On the outside of the card, Leo had drawn a picture of a man lying in a bed. The caption under it read, "My dad had to go to the hospital." Inside the card was a picture of a man standing and smiling with the caption, "But he didn't die."

It was difficult for me to look at cards like that one. First of all, it bothered me that I remembered so little of the days leading up to and immediately following my cardiac arrest. But thinking of the event from the perspective of Leo and the rest of my family, I felt guilty that what I had gone through caused such trauma for them. I guess what troubled me the most was that I couldn't shake the dread I felt from almost dying and leaving them behind.

Like most married men my age, I suspect, I'd never imagined myself not being around to see my kids grow up or my wife's hair turn grey along with mine. I'd never thought about Debbie having to place a claim on my life insurance to pay the mortgage and the bills so that she could stay home to raise our children on her own. I looked around the house at the state I'd left it in and shook my head: income tax receipts in a dozen different places that Debbie would never have been able to find; a dangling light bulb hanging from the ceiling of our bedroom, replacing a fixture I had removed to try and fix; my desk covered in unlabeled files; my workbench awash in dozens of unsorted screws and bolts. I shuddered at how unprepared I was.

But can we ever be prepared? There were no warning signs for me: no chest pains or shortness of breath. I was simply running in a race, as I had several times before. I must have been struggling, but I don't remember how I felt. Ron Youngash, who started administering the CPR, said I collapsed suddenly. I didn't slowly buckle. And without the chest compressions and ventilation I received, I would have died right there: my income tax undone, my desk covered in various files, and my bedroom lighted by a bare bulb. "Like a thief in the night," the Bible describes the suddenness of death. And so it could have been for me.

*How do we know when it's time
to make changes in our lives?*

Looking at Leo's card, I realized that I was becoming more aware of this suddenness. And I'd tried to make changes. I hadn't cleaned my desk or workbench, and I hadn't fixed the light fixture in my bedroom. But I had begun to reach out more. I wasn't as quick to anger with my children. I hugged them more and I tried to listen to them more. I tried to listen to my wife as well. My recovery involved steadily lengthening daily walks that we usually took together, talking the whole time. We hugged more too. I saw my friends more often. Many of them dropped by. Others called. Sometimes I even ventured out to visit them. And we hugged as well.

I now knew where my heart was. It was right behind the scar that ran down my chest to my belly. Even though it sometimes hurt to grasp someone to it, I felt compelled to hug the friends and family I saw. And I thought they felt the same way. They saw in me the preciousness and fragility of life. By pressing against the wired-together rib cage that enclosed my triple-bypassed heart, maybe they felt they could understand that preciousness themselves, and know my heart was not just behind that rib cage, but within them as well.

I hoped they could.

Thinking about what it would have been like for my family had I died was the hardest part. I would have wanted to have said my goodbyes to them or at least have written something to each of them. I'd written about all of them in columns and articles over the years, but I didn't write to them enough.

After my grandmother died several years ago, my father gave my sisters and me a photocopy of a note she'd written. It wasn't long. She wrote it for everyone: her children, her grandchildren and her great grandchildren. Yet it meant a great deal to me. It began, "To my darlings. Just in case." In the few, short sentences that followed, she gave her love to all of us. It was a simple note, but one I cherished.

I began to compose a letter to my own family. Just in case.

21

ON BECOMING NICE

"Why are you so nice now?" Leo asked me one day for no apparent reason.

"What do you mean now?" I asked.

"Now, since you were in the hospital about your heart."

I didn't know how to respond. I just hugged him and kissed him on the head saying, "Thanks for saying that."

When I thought about his comments later, though, I was both pleased and saddened – pleased that I'd changed, but sad because Leo obviously thought that I hadn't always been such a nice guy.

That was one of the positive outcomes of everything I'd gone through since January 11th. I was nicer, I guess. I rarely lost my temper. I loved spending time with Debbie and the kids. And I had more opportunity to reflect on what was most important in life.

Can personalities change?

Like many families I know, we've developed a traditional seating arrangement around our dinner table. We have a large, formal dining room in our home. In the middle of the room stands a hefty, oak table we bought second hand many years ago. With the three leaves in it, the table can seat 12 people. I've always sat at one end of the table. I guess it's the head of the table since it's closest to the built-in buffet where we often place the food we're serving and the closest to the kitchen.

As we gathered to sit for dinner one evening shortly after I had arrived home from the hospital, I was suddenly struck by the realization that I didn't know whether I should be sitting at the head of the table. My mom was still staying with us. Keith and Luanne had come over for dinner, just as they probably had many times while I was in the hospital. For all those dinners my family had shared, someone else had sat at the head of the table. I didn't know if a new pattern had developed, but I felt that I didn't really deserve to be sitting there. I felt like an interloper, someone crashing the party, not the head of the family.

I sensed hesitation in Keith as well, and realized that he had probably been the one to sit in my place. Of course, he and everyone else insisted that I sit in my customary place. Still, I felt oddly out of place. Like Macbeth wearing the kingly robes of the slain Duncan, I felt ill suited for my position.

To a certain degree, that misplaced feeling remained with me for some time. For several weeks, I bowed to Debbie's control of the household. I was too weak to do much – too tired to bring myself to any kind of position of parental authority. I'd never regarded myself as the authority figure in the household, but I often felt powerless in many ways. One day, I quizzed Debbie about how I appeared to her.

"You're quieter," she said, "and gentler."

I was quiet. I rarely raised my voice. I let Debbie deal with any family conflicts that developed. Sometimes I felt like less of a father and husband and more a visitor.

Is everyone searching for new ways to find meaning?

I remember having coffee with a friend around the same time as Leo had made his comment. My friend talked about wanting to find more meaning in his life, just as I wanted to understand what the events of these last three months were meant to tell me. I felt relieved that I had decided not to jump back into the teaching fray immediately. I wasn't ready to do that. The stress and exhaustion I had felt recently, while interviewing for and writing a magazine article, showed me how low my energy level truly was. Like my friend, I sensed I was meant to do more. I'd found fulfillment in teaching, but I felt compelled to do something else as well. I wasn't even sure that writing was it. Even though I didn't sit down every-day to jot down my thoughts, books had been the centre of much of my life and I'd always thought of myself as some sort of writer.

After Leo's birth, I spent most of my days in the next few years caring for him at home and working as a freelance journalist. I tried to maintain the habit of mailing at least one manuscript or article proposal a week. But after months of trying, I still hadn't sold a story. The arrival of the mail everyday, nonetheless, was a hugely anticipated event for Leo and me. At least it was for me.

One day the mail arrived as usual and, carrying Leo in one arm, I retrieved a magazine, a couple of bills and one of the

familiar self-addressed stamped envelopes I sent with every proposal. Still holding Leo, I tore open the envelope anticipating another of the many polite rejection letters I'd received. As I pulled
a folded letter from the envelope, though, a smaller piece of paper
fell to the floor. I glanced down at what looked amazingly like a
cheque. Shaking, I sat in a chair, Leo on my lap, and read the letter
in my hands.

"Thank you for your submission. Please find enclosed a cheque
in payment for your story...."

I couldn't read the rest. The story was about my grandfather.
It was set in my grandparents' apartment at Christmas and was
based on memories of my childhood and his recollections of the
war. I'd sent it to a small magazine in the United States that, my
research had shown, published similar stories. Tears flowed down
my cheeks as I hugged Leo and as images and memories of my
grandfather flooded through me.

After my heart attack, it had taken me several weeks to success-
fully put pen to paper. I'd tried to write as early as when I was
hospitalized, but my scrawled sentences were even difficult for me
to decipher. I feared my oxygen-deprived brain wouldn't work as
it once had. I feared the same thing with writing a book. Could I
really do it? Did I want to risk failing?

Like other sudden death experiences I'd read about, mine had
given me a chance to reinvent my entire life. This was a new life
for me. I really did have two birthdays now: the day I was born
and the day I was reborn after my heart stopped on a country
road. And I should be able to do whatever I wanted with my

second life. In some ways, I was waiting for the same kind of lightning bolts that had struck Dannion Brinkley and Gretel Ehrlich. I had recently read both of their memoirs in which they each wrote about their near-death experiences after being struck by lightning. They seemed to have reached profound understandings of their places in the world as a result of their experiences. The lightning strikes had jolted them into a new reality. Dannion Brinkley began to care for dying war veterans and Gretel Ehrlich has traveled through Greenland and the Arctic writing about the indigenous peoples in those regions and the consequences of climate change on their environments.

But I didn't need to wait for my own lightning bolt. I'd already been struck. When the jolt to my heart from the defibrillator administered by the ambulance attendants brought my heartbeat back to a regular rhythm, I also came back. I just needed to see the light that journey had created and find my own way of writing about it.

22

SIMPLY LET GO

"So are you going to keep running now?" Dr. Michael Greenwood asked me.

"Sure, I probably will."

"Why would you want to do that? It killed you."

After thinking about it for a few days, I had finally decided to go back to see Dr. Greenwood for an acupuncture treatment. Before he began his treatment, insisting I call him Michael, he talked about a discussion we'd had in our previous session. He'd asked about how I perceived my normal body temperature, and I told him that I often felt cold. My hands and feet were always cold, actually. He then suggested my running might be a quick fix to warm my body up. It was a temporary solution, though, since, just as quickly, I'd cool down after running. We concentrated on what drove me to run.

Running had always been a form of fitness for me and I'd never thought of it as something I was driven to do. Many of the runners in the races I often ran in were driven, but I didn't think

I was like that. Yet he called running an addiction for me – especially running in races.

"I really don't feel as though I'm addicted to running," I said.

"All addicts deny they're addicts," he said with a sly smile.

There was some truth to what Michael said. My cardiologist, Dr. Morgan, had suggested that I could continue running, but that I probably shouldn't run to the same level that I had in the past.

"You don't want to be a martyr," he said.

When I told Michael about my cardiologist's comments, he said, "Those with an imbalance towards coldness, as you have, are often martyrs."

I hadn't thought of myself as a martyr either. Yet there had been something driving me since the event. I liked the idea that I was out of the hospital four days after the bypass operation. I had this competitive desire to be better than the average. If it took most people a week to recover in the hospital after heart surgery, I had to be out sooner. I had read, recently, that sedentary workers could be back at work 4 to 6 weeks after surgery. That bothered me. It made me think that I should have returned to teaching right away.

As I started to walk with Michael into the acupuncture treatment room, he suggested that I should "write and write and write." He wasn't suggesting high levels of production, but he was encouraging me to set the groundwork for a quest. "Cold people are often on a quest," he told me, "but they don't often know what that quest is. They're searching, but they're often doing it blind."

Was I really addicted to running?

Michael had given me a great deal to think about. I'd often worried about having an addictive personality. I tended to throw myself completely into an endeavour. Perhaps running had been like that. I liked to think of it as simply exercise: something to keep me fit, an activity that gave me a regular endorphin rush but wasn't condemned by society or considered illegal. To me, running was a socially sanctioned high I was able to achieve three or four times a week simply by putting on a pair of running shoes, some shorts and a t-shirt, then loping through the streets for 45 minutes.

But was running an addictive activity? My parents and sisters weren't runners. In fact their lifestyles were very different from the one I'd adopted. My parents smoked as I was growing up and continued to until very recently. My father says a letter he received from Raechel urging him to quit was the catalyst for his finally stopping. He's struggled with drinking all of his adult life as well, but rarely overdrinks today. He now has control over his vices. Do I have control over mine?

And what about the martyr in me? When I finally began to understand what had happened after my cardiac arrest, I would spend hours reading the many cards and letters that friends and family had sent. Friends from my childhood phoned and even visited just to tell me they were happy to hear or see me alive. At times, I felt like Tom Sawyer hiding in the church choir loft and listening to the eulogy at his own funeral. I liked that attention. And at some level, I think I liked the fact that people were feeling sorry for me. Was I pushing myself into unwitting martyrdom simply to feel that again?

Why would someone agree to have needles pushed into his skin?

When we reached Michael's treatment room, he asked me to lie down on a covered mattress on the floor. "As you'll find out," he said, "it makes more sense to have my treatment area on the floor rather than an elevated table." He knelt on the carpeted floor next to me, lit what seemed to me to be a piece of incense, and then placed it on the inside of my wrist. "Let me know when you feel this," he said.

Almost immediately, I felt a sharp burning pain. "I feel it," I blurted, and he quickly wiped something off my wrist. He explained that he was warming up the pressure points and carried out the same procedure on other parts of my hands and arms, wiping off the heated incense just before the pain became too great.

As I closed my eyes, I couldn't see exactly what he was doing, but I became aware that Michael had begun to arrange the tools of his trade, the needles, next to my body. I breathed deeply, trying to relax.

Suddenly, I felt a sharpness pierce my skin as Michael inserted a needle into a pressure point near my wrist. The feeling wasn't painful, just slightly uncomfortable. As he pushed the needle in further, I felt a slight electrical shock jolt me. The shock didn't emanate from outside my body, but stemmed from within, stimulated by the probing needles. I sank further into the mattress lying on the floor of his treatment room.

I began to breathe deeply as Michael inserted more needles. He had encouraged me to vocalize, as loudly as I could, when I exhaled. With each breath, I cried out, first in gentle murmurs, but soon in loud moans.

Michael continued to insert needles and encourage my vocalizations: "Great. Those sounds are terrific."

Then my voice changed. I began to sound like I was singing a long, extended "ahh" each time I breathed out.

"Keep singing," he said.

I tried to keep the vocalizations going, my voice getting louder as I continued to sing. With each deep breath and each exhalation, I produced a different tone, a different note. Encouraged by Michael, I continued to increase the volume of the sounds until they were no longer notes, but wails, the sounds coming from somewhere deep within my body. Soon the wails turned to sobs as I started to cry uncontrollably.

"That's it," called Michael above the sound of my cries. "Let it come."

Becoming exhausted by the emotional release, I felt my sobs begin to subside as Michael moved down my body continuing to insert needles. When he reached my ankles, my body began to shake. He encouraged me to move even more. As he inserted a needle near the instep of my right foot, my whole body quivered. My legs started to bounce on the mattress as I began to lose complete control of my limbs.

"Good. Keep moving," he encouraged me.

The shaking moved up my legs to my pelvis. Soon, my whole lower body was quaking. Michael grabbed my shoulders as my body started to shake off the mattress.

After pulling me back to the centre of the mattress, Michael moved up towards my torso. My eyes were closed, but I was aware of his hands as he placed them over my chest. His hands hovered over me, not quite touching the left side of my sternum where the pain and numbness of the heart surgery was still strong.

Before his hands touched me, however, my chest began to bounce up off the mattress. My body reacted as it must have when the defibrillator paddles were placed on me. My chest jolted upward several times.

Slowly, my head started to move back and forth. The pillow that was under my head had long since slipped off the mattress, but I began to rhythmically shake my head from one side to the other, hitting the side of my face against the mattress each time.

As my head moved, the shaking in my legs began to change. My legs started to bounce against the mattress one after the other in a rhythmic motion. Soon my arms began to move in the same pattern. At my side, they banged against the mattress in alternating thrusts. I suddenly realized that I was running. I was lying on my back, on a mattress on the floor, with my eyes closed. But I was running.

Michael encouraged the movement. If I began to slow down, he gently rocked my head back and forth again. I was breathing hard. I felt sweat begin to run down my forehead. I was exhausted. But I continued to run.

My eyes still closed, I began to see images. In my mind, I pictured, for the first time, the end of the eight-kilometre race that culminated in my cardiac arrest. I saw the gravel road leading to the finish. I was aware of the banner across the road marking the finish line itself. I strained as I ran up the hill. My breathing had increased. My mouth agape, I tried to suck in more air as I laboured up the hill toward the finish.

I reached the line. And I collapsed.

My body stopped moving. All around me, I saw blackness. I was aware of nothing but that blackness as I sank slowly into it, deeper and deeper.

How much of the race
did I actually see?

When I thought about the acupuncture treatment later, it wasn't hard for me to see parallels between the night terrors I had as a child and the black void I descended into during Michael's treatment. But I felt no terror with Michael. Even as the movements of my body seemed to take on the cadences of a runner and I was able to actually visualize the ending of the race, I felt no fear. The lack of fear surprised me, as did the depths to which I was able to enter into the treatment and the complete trust I had of Michael's abilities to guide me. I had met him only twice, but felt completely at ease with him.

Michael called his treatment deep acupuncture. The experience was certainly deep for me. I had thought about having a hypnosis treatment to try to bring back the memories of the race, but

Michael's acupuncture had done just that even though I was not expecting it to. Reliving the experience, even at this level, helped me. I felt no pain. I felt no fear. I crossed the finish line again. And simply let go.

23

THE MANY BENEFITS
OF RUNNING

"For me, the benefits of running are simple," I told the crowd of runners. "If I hadn't been a runner, the collateral arteries wouldn't have formed around my blocked arteries. I probably would have had a heart attack while eating nachos or watching reruns of *Seinfeld*. Chances are, there wouldn't have been any doctors around. Running was a lifeline for me."

Not long after the bypass surgery, I spoke to about 550 people who had competed in a five-kilometre race at the university. I was supposed to talk about the benefits of running, but knowing that many of the same people who had been at the Harriers 8K would be at this race, I wanted to publicly thank them, especially those who had helped me at the race. Ron Youngash, Dan Baker, Rachel Staples, and Cheryl Wood were all there.

I met Ron for the first time that day. At least it was the first time that I consciously remember meeting him. He came up to me after the speech to congratulate me and to say hello. As soon as I saw him, I knew who he was. His face was immediately familiar to me. When I shook his hand, a memory of him as he was doing CPR on me flashed through my mind. It was a startling feeling to see him and to realize that I remembered him on some level.

The talk went well. The crowd didn't overwhelm me. I felt that I was able to say what I had wanted to say and do it without being overly emotional. I had feared that I might break down in tears in the middle of the talk – that the emotions running through me would be too much to handle. I had written a complete speech, but I didn't have to look at my notes. I spoke directly to the crowd and offered my thanks. It was a big step for me.

Why is it so hard to believe in miracles?

John Catterall, the man who led the prayers over my unconscious body at the race, was there as well. He told me that he was speaking the next evening at his church as part of a course about miracles. He asked me if I could attend and speak with him. Hesitating slightly, I decided to go. My hesitation wasn't based on my not acknowledging the miracle that my healing was and continued to be. I just wasn't sure about acknowledging it in front of dozens of people. That was another big step for me. I felt that I wanted to give hope. Speaking at the race seemed to offer that hope for people I'd never met before. Many runners came up to me to say how positive it was for them to see me up and functioning. I felt offering that hope was important, and I felt privileged being able to do it. But most of all I wanted to thank everyone. That was my primary motivation in speaking at the race. Being some sort of role model for runners was secondary. Now John was asking me to be part of something that could lead to being a role model for the power of miracles as well. That was decidedly different.

I had never been to John's church. I knew of it as a somewhat evangelical congregation, a church that would welcome the presence of two people involved in a miracle. Debbie and I went together and we sat with John as the church's minister talked about the reality of miracles in our lives. At the end of his talk, he introduced John and me as embodiments of what he had been talking about. John and I stood up in front of the more than 50 people there that evening and began to tell our story. It was really John's story and he did most of the speaking. He told about reluctantly missing church that Sunday because he felt strangely compelled to run the race. He told about wearing the bright red Jesus shirt under a thicker sweatshirt. He told about his trepidation in praying for me in front of a crowd and the greater nervousness in asking strangers to join in with him. I was really his prop. He told the story, and I was the living embodiment of what he saw as a miraculous result of his story.

I did say a few words that evening. Unlike when I spoke to the running community, I didn't boisterously acknowledge my fighting spirit to survive and run again. To this audience, I talked about the power of prayer and the strength in belief. I told them I believe that miracles occur around us everyday, but that we're not always ready to see or acknowledge them. I said that, for me, John's presence and intervention at the race were just as important to my survival as were the actions of the doctors who performed CPR.

Do psychics see more than we do?

Although I'd attended church in the past, visiting John's church and its overt evangelicalism was a new experience for me. I had another new, almost churchlike experience some time later when I attended a lecture given by Sylvia Browne. She's a famous psychic I'd never heard of until I saw an ad in the paper advertising her lecture. For some reason, I felt as though I should go hear her speak.

I didn't know it when I first saw the ad, but two friends of mine, Charlene and Jenny, had already bought tickets to see her. They had gone to see a palm reader who told them that they should attend her lecture and should take a friend. They immediately sensed that I was the friend. I decided to look into buying a ticket, but found that the presentation was sold out. Then two days before the lecture, Jenny called to say that her husband couldn't go to the lecture so she had an extra ticket. Debbie was a bit worried about the idea of my going to see a psychic and looked up several websites about Sylvia Browne, some of which presented her in a less than flattering manner. My misgivings grew.

The night before her talk, I had trouble sleeping as I mulled over everything. Despite what seemed like positive signs leading me towards attending the event, I still had concerns about going. I did go, however, meeting Jenny and Charlene outside the theatre just before the 8 o'clock show.

The theatre was packed with over 1,200 people, mostly women, I noticed. A prompter was on stage when we arrived trying to whip the crowd into a frenzy. We found our seats and started crawling over several pairs of legs when we learned that we should have picked up tickets for a draw to choose the few who would be given the chance to ask questions of Sylvia in the second half of the show. I gave my entrance ticket to Jenny so she could claim my draw ticket. She returned with three tickets, handed one to each of us, and we once again took our seats.

When the lights dimmed, a man came on stage and quickly, but exuberantly, introduced Sylvia Browne. A bleached-blonde woman in her sixties walked across the stage to an armchair and microphone placed downstage centre. She sat in the chair, and for over an hour, regaled us with stories and tales revealing her theories along the way. I was surprised at her wit and cynicism. She was more like a stand up comic seated in an easy chair than a renowned psychic. She believes in angels, Spirit guides and the power of God's love. Earth is the true hell, she thinks. Passing over to the other side is what we long for, but we don't always get to stay there. We live many lives, coming back to figure out the right way to live each time. It's a theory that obviously struck home for many in the audience who would burst into applause every few minutes and even gave her a couple of standing ovations before the first half was over.

The second half began with a briefer lecture followed by a guided meditation that she led. Then she started drawing numbers. I had read on one of the websites that Debbie looked at about the process her lectures typically go through. So I had imagined my getting the chance to ask her a question. Of course, I thought of asking her about my cardiac arrest. In fact, under my collared shirt, I wore the Harriers 8K t-shirt that had been given to me after the race. It's a shirt I rarely ever wore, but for some reason, I felt compelled to wear it that night.

Then it happened. The numbers were drawn. When I checked my ticket stub, I moaned.

"What's wrong?" Jenny asked.

"My number."

"You're number was chosen?" asked Charlene.

"Do you want it?" I asked.

"Of course not."

"Here, Jenny you take it."

"Greg, your number was chosen. It's yours. That's so exciting."

Charlene and Jenny were thrilled about the evening and they both so longed to ask Sylvia a question that I wanted one of them to have the chance. Jenny had arbitrarily handed us our draw tickets. Why should this one be mine? I slumped in my chair, not wanting to get up and move to one of the two microphones set up for the questions. Finally, after more encouragement from Jenny and Charlene, I did move and made my way to the end of one of the lines.

As I inched closer to the microphone, I considered what I should ask, wondering if I could bring up a question that Jenny and Charlene would have wanted to pose. Finally I reached the microphone, and decided to combine the two ideas. I began by saying that I was here with two friends who had been told by a palm reader that they should go see Sylvia Browne and to take me along. I wondered why they would have received such a message, especially concerning me since I had experienced a cardiac arrest, been virtually dead for twenty minutes, and now wondered what my reintroduction to life meant.

Sylvia went for the laugh first, saying that she had paid the palm reader. After the laughs subsided, she continued to say that a feeling of warmth and love was what we should be experiencing here. But the question of my rebirth was more important. She said that I was meant to come back to life. The fact that I wasn't brain dead when I should have been was evidence enough of the message I needed to express.

"You're a walking experience of what I say," she went on. "If you're not supposed to go, you won't go. So that was your exit point and you just didn't want to go. But what you should do is write. Seriously."

I was dumbfounded. I couldn't help feeling that everything had fallen into place, as it should have: that I was meant to be there and was meant to hear that message. Her responses to the questions were usually safe and general. But when she told me that I had to write, I felt that she was tapping into exactly what was important for me. Her message to me was vital – even life changing.

Is the understanding
of spirituality a personal quest?

My personal spirituality was different than both John's and Sylvia's, however. It had grown from my childhood Catholicism, from "my lost saints" that were like those Elizabeth Barrett

Browning refers to in her famous poem. The ecumenism that Father Leo had embodied affected me. So had my travels.

My visit to Rome had given me a new impression of the historical Catholic Church. Traveling through Britain later, I was exposed to a belief system and a mythology that were even older. From Bath to Tintagel, from Glastonbury Abbey to Exeter Cathedral, I began to come to an understanding of the interconnectedness of Ancient Rome, Celtic mythology and Christianity. The mythical King Arthur, conceived at Tintagel, was born a bastard, the son of King Uther and Ygraine. Like Jesus Christ, he was born into a world of strife, but born as a pauper, not a king. Jesus, too, was born to an unmarried Mary and Joseph. He was ironically named the King of the Jews at his death, but he united the Christian world from a position of weakness, just as Arthur united the British world from a position of weakness.

These saviours of the world are purposefully not entrenched in the world. They are otherworldly, not caught up in the affairs of the temporal. Their strengths come from their weaknesses. Just as Ghandi's power to overthrow British rule in India came from passivity not violence.

I was more moved seeing Tintagel and Stonehenge than I had been seeing Rome as a nineteen-year-old. The simplicity of Stonehenge, the mystery of Tintagel meant more to me than the opulence of the Vatican because of the spirit they embody not the grandeur.

Health issues leave us in positions of weakness as well. As we heal, we're forced to reflect and take stock. Because we're battling a force attempting to control from within, we can no longer look outward towards external battles. We have to look inward. My heart disease diagnosis gave me the opportunity to examine the path I was following, to evaluate my life, and to heal. From that illness, a supposed state of weakness, I'd been given the power to move forward, the strength to overcome, and the knowledge that comes with reflection.

24

DEALING WITH A BRAIN INJURY

"Now Gregory Marchand," my neighbour Leslie called from across the street. "Are you sure you should be climbing that ladder?"

A mother, a teacher, and a wife, Leslie knew well the chastising power of using someone's full name. By that point she had crossed the street and was standing beneath the ladder I had just climbed up to the second storey of our house.

My recovery at home after my cardiac surgery went through many phases. The physical recovery was gradual but steady. I walked: first half a block, then the full length of the street, then around the block entirely. Gradually my walks became blocks, and eventually miles. I slowly pushed myself walking, trying to gauge how hard my heart was working, but slowing down when I felt tired.

I tried to re-immerse myself in household routines as well. Sitting in the living room one day in early spring, I had looked out the window to realize that our outdoor Christmas lights were still up. Their presence became a nagging concern for me knowing that Debbie wouldn't feel comfortable climbing a ladder to take them down. After she had gone out that afternoon, I hauled the ladder out from the basement, leaned it against the house, and started to climb. Before I had even reached out to grasp the first string of bulbs, I heard a voice calling from across the street. Leslie was the same friend who had first taken Debbie to the hospital the day I collapsed.

From atop the ladder, I looked down at Leslie and smiled. "Thanks for looking after me, Gladys Kravitz," I said, knowing she'd understand the 1960s *Bewitched* allusion.

"Well, someone has to. I saw Debbie leave and then you come around with the ladder right away. Why don't I ask Dave to come over and take them down when he gets home from work?"

I appreciated Leslie's offering her husband's assistance, but I felt the need to try doing this on my own. "The longer these stay up, the lower the neighbourhood's property values plummet," I said grinning.

"Okay, okay. But I'm going to be over there watching you just in case. Be careful."

"Don't worry, Leslie. I will."

I was careful. In fact it took me twice as long to take them down as I had imagined, and I was exhausted by the time I finished. I felt rejuvenated, though. I had accomplished something.

Will my brain ever
function the same way again?

Accomplishments were slow in coming, especially when they required some sort of mental effort. I was finding that my brain was moving at a much slower pace than I wanted it to. I was in the midst of reading a book I'd taken out of the library. I loved Mordechai Richler's writing and was enjoying his novel, *Barney's Version*. Reading it wasn't easy, however. I found myself having to re-read entire passages when a plot development made no sense to me. Characters seemed to pop into the story out of nowhere, until I looked back to see that they had been introduced pages earlier.

Numbers seemed to be even more of a problem to me. I had always completed Debbie's and my income tax returns myself and as this year's filing deadline approached, worked at making sense of the receipts and forms piled on my desk. The work was even more tedious than ever, but I knew that persevering through it would help the healing going on in my brain. My pride in completing the task well before the deadline was short-lived when I received a reply from the taxation department reassessing both returns because of simple arithmetical errors.

I continued to struggle with the nature of my brain injury when I eventually started teaching part-time. In less than a year, I had gone from a hospital patient who couldn't remember how old he was to a teacher passing on the finer points of writing and literature to students who unquestioningly trusted his knowledge.

Does a drop in cognitive ability increase empathy?

One day I was working with a former student of mine who had also suffered a brain injury several years previously. I had taught her when she was in grade 10, about a decade earlier. Now, she was still taking a grade 10 math course in a school for adult learners. Ironically, I was helping out in the Learning Resource Centre and was trying to help her with her math, the subject area I felt least comfortable with since my own brain injury. She was as charming and vivacious as she had been a decade before, seemingly oblivious to the fact that she hadn't advanced in her studies despite 10 years of trying. She talked about finishing her course work in order to go on to university to study veterinary medicine, the same goal she had when I taught her previously.

But when I tried to help her with her grade 10 math problem, her struggles and frustrations became apparent. She became embarrassed after asking me a question about why her answer didn't match the answer key and then discovered that she had written the problem down incorrectly. She seemed to see her struggle as a fault of her own.

I saw it differently. I knew what was going on in her mind because I'd had the same feelings. I'd wondered whether my comments made any sense to anyone but me. I'd questioned whether someone I'd been talking to had walked away thinking, "Poor guy. He's just not completely there anymore." And I'd apologized for my lapses in memory or understanding, embarrassed by my shortcomings just as my student now was.

I truly empathized with her. I saw her struggling to form the words to explain a problem she was facing, knowing that within her brain, the explanation was clear but her ability to transfer that expression to her lips was faulty. She knew it was faulty, but she couldn't even articulate that knowledge. Instead, she laughed in frustration in front of me and probably cried when she got home.

My struggle was similar. Sometimes, I was afraid to push far enough to try and understand how much my brain had been impaired. I taught a limited amount without branching into courses that might challenge me to learn more. I wrote about safe subjects avoiding issues that I might have to debate.

Debate scared me. I was never sure whether my mind was keeping up with the discussion whenever I fell into conversation with a group of people. I wondered if my comments had relevance. I got lost trying to formulate my views on a particular point that had been raised only to find that point had been long surpassed by the time I was ready to add my views. I felt as though I was traveling two or three steps behind everyone else.

Yet I wasn't really sure whether my feelings were accurate or not. I'd read that brain injury patients both deny the effects of their injuries and blame a host of problems on them. Was I placing blame where it didn't belong? Was I fooling myself into believing that I actually had the capacity to teach meaningfully? I didn't know the answers. I stumbled along, questioning my actions, my thoughts, and my abilities, all the while fearful that I might wake up one morning unable to remember how old I was again.

25

RUNNING WITH LUCAS

"Are you ready to give me CPR if I collapse?" I asked Lucas. "Don't even say that," he said.

Lucas and I had gone out for a run together almost six months after my cardiac arrest. It was the first run I'd attempted since then. Of course, I'd thought a great deal about running. The act of running itself was so much part of my life that I couldn't possibly give it up entirely. I had filled myself with positive memories of running: the smell of damp leaves on a chip trail in the fall, the sun breaking over the horizon so that I'd have to suddenly squint running along a deserted road in the morning, the pride in pulling off a completely sweat-soaked shirt after a mid-summer jaunt, the winter air filling my lungs, the rhythmic slap of my running shoes on the late night street, the salty ocean breeze on my face.

Yet I knew that I had to run differently now. I knew that running could no longer be a competitive pursuit for me, that it should be more contemplative, more recreational, more a source of exercise. I also knew that I couldn't run alone. Although running had largely been a solitary endeavor for me, the one person who could truly be called my running partner was Lucas.

Lucas and I ran for about 25 minutes, passing an ambulance along the way, its siren wailing. We ran through the parking lot of my cardiologist's office. We even ran by the hospital where my surgery had taken place and where my heart had been intentionally stopped a second time. I was aware of my heart the whole time we were running. Several times, I noticed Lucas glancing at my sweating, reddening face with concern.

My heart felt fine. My legs hurt. My shirt was soaked in sweat. But I felt fine.

We walked up the final hill towards our house calling it a warm down. Without saying anything to each other, we both were aware that pushing up the final hill was exactly how I'd collapsed on January 11th. We didn't want to force this first run too much. When we reached the crest of the hill, Lucas reached over, patted me on the back and said, "That was great."

Times had changed. In all the runs we'd done together to that point, I had been the encourager. I was the one to offer the supportive pat on the back. In the middle of our run, he had looked over, and down, at me and said, "I hadn't realized until now how much taller than you I am." I couldn't remember the last time we'd run together, but I was sure I was the taller one then.

Now he was. He was tall in stature and tall in his support. I couldn't have run like that on my own. I felt confident running with Lucas. It was entirely appropriate that he was the one I should run with for the first time. We'd always run together. Running had been our wordless means of communication. I was his first running coach and had watched him win City and Island running championships. And now he was the one supporting my attempt to return to running.

Was it really my heart that made me so emotional?

I'd read that heart patients often experience an increased sensitivity to events in their lives. Emotionally, we're often on the edge and feel those emotions more acutely than we did previously. I found that I was often quick to tears. I worried about being in emotionally charged situations, fearing that my reactions would embarrass me and those around me.

At Lucas' school awards night that spring, I found myself caught in that sort of situation. For two days prior to the awards presentations, we had three different phone calls from the school letting us know that Lucas would be receiving something. One caller "strongly urged" us to attend with other family members. So I was anticipating an emotional night.

When his PE teacher launched into a lengthy monologue in praise of the still unidentified winner of the boys' Athletic Award, I tried to keep track of his comments thinking the winner might be Lucas. By the time he ended his preamble saying, "And no one should be prouder than you, Mr. and Mrs. Marchand," I was sobbing.

When the principal then began his tribute to the winner of the Leadership Award, I was already an emotional wreck. His description of the recipient leading up to the announcement of the winner soon made it obvious that this award was going to Lucas as well. Sitting beside me, Raechel kept poking me in the ribs amusingly embarrassed at my reaction. When the lights were finally turned on at the end of the presentations, I casually tried to wipe my eyes before anyone noticed my tear-stained face.

After the run with Lucas, I wondered how much I'd run in the future. I didn't know if running was still the right form of exercise for me. I'd established a peacefulness in my life that the walking and yoga I was doing supported and encouraged. I wondered if running would undermine that peace. But I also realized that attitude was the truly important factor. Lucas and I weren't running to compete. We were running to support. And his support had given me strength to choose any type of activity I wanted.

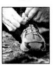

26

CONTEMPLATIVE
ACUPUNCTURE

"I've been thinking a lot about death," I told Michael Greenwood.

"That's not surprising," he said. "You've come as close to death without passing over as anyone I've met."

"When I think about that, I realize how easy it would be to just go back."

"Well, don't worry. No one's ever died during one of my treatments."

I was back to see Dr. Michael Greenwood for another acupuncture treatment after several weeks of regaining strength and health. The only time I could book with him, however, turned out to be the day before a party we had been planning to thank everyone who had been involved in my collapse and recovery. I had been a little worried about the treatment, remembering how exhausted I was after the first one and anticipating the emotional energy I would likely be expending at the party the next day. I had spent much of Thursday morning getting ready for the party including cutting the lawn, the first time I'd done anything that strenuous since January 11th. By the time I got to Michael's clinic at 2 pm, I was already a little tired.

As Michael went through the process of warming the acupuncture points, he continued to talk on the theme of death. Michael said that he views death as a journey or process. He thinks that the Western world ascribes too much fear to that process. I understood what he was saying. When I think about my own death, I'm not as concerned about myself as much as about those I'd leave behind. During our first acupuncture session when I began to sob, I was thinking about the impact on my family and friends of the preceding weeks, not about my own fears. There have been times since I've been home that I've even felt almost welcoming towards the idea of death. Especially in the first few weeks, I keenly felt the burdens of everyday life. I had a hard time coping with the simple tasks of washing dishes and putting Leo to bed and found myself overly concerned about the more profound issues of environmental degradation and global warming. Even thinking of the day-to-day process of making a living worried me. Sometimes, death felt easier. Without my family to think about, death might have been welcoming.

At the end of the treatment, I fell into a deep meditation, much deeper than I do with my daily meditations. I was within the blackness of the void we had talked about, that he had written about in one of his books, that I had experienced during my childhood terrors, and that I had slipped into during the previous session. Then the blackness began to change.

Can healing occur spontaneously?

The day before, I had received a phone call from a woman I hadn't heard from for several years. She had been the general manager of Butchart Gardens the five years I had performed in the summer stage show there. She had gone to school with Debbie, and I remembered her as an organized, capable manager. That day, she had read a magazine piece I'd written about my illness while waiting for her daughter in a dentist's office and was calling to see how I was doing. She said she was concerned about my well being, but was curious about what I had gone through because of the work she was now doing. She explained that she had been channeling information to people through writing. She didn't know how or why it worked, but she felt she had been able to help a number of people understand problems and move in new directions in their lives. It sounded a little strange, but I was interested in what she was doing and impressed with her sincerity. As we were saying goodbye, she advised me to try to visualize the colour green when meditating since green is a healing colour.

The next two times I meditated, I did try to visualize green with no success. But in the middle of the deep meditation after Michael's treatment, the blackness I saw suddenly began to change. I pictured a series of green, moving circles. For several minutes, I watched them move then surround me. I felt as though my body were plunging through the circles themselves. It was a warming, relaxing experience.

In the midst of this, I began to become aware of Michael moving. I knew that my time must have been almost up, but I couldn't pull myself completely into consciousness. Finally, I was able to open my eyes. He was beside me smiling, but I could barely keep my eyes focused to smile back. I tried to talk but felt like I was drifting. It reminded me of the medication-induced haze I had been in when I was in the hospital.

Slowly, my voice slurred, "I feel like I'm on morphine."

He laughed gently, placed a blanket on me and told me I could remain there for longer if I wanted. He left the room saying, "Just let that morphine drip work."

For some time, I did just that. I tried to let myself go further, to allow the healing green circles to surround me even more. I felt myself drift deeper into the mattress as my surroundings disappeared and the warmth of my visualizations increased, relaxing me even more. The blackness I'd descended into earlier in the treatment had been replaced with a warm light from which the circles of green emanated. The more I drifted, the lighter I felt, and the brighter my surroundings became. I felt blissfully relaxed and utterly contented.

The sudden call of a gull outside brought me back to reality and Michael's treatment room. I was completely unaware of the time that had passed, but sensed I was over my allotted hour and didn't want to take advantage of Michael. As I had in the hospital, I felt the need to fight against the haze, so forced myself to open my eyes, slowly shaking my head against the mattress and beginning to stretch my legs.

Finally, I was able to stand up, put my socks and shoes on, and walk to Michael's office. By that time I was quite alert. In fact, I felt rested and rejuvenated. Michael was excited about the process. He had recognized that in my movements and shaking during the treatment, I was running as I had done the first time. And he knew that the 20-minute meditation I'd experienced following the treatment was a healing process for me. Because of that process, he told me that he didn't think that I would have to come back. He said I could if I wanted, but he felt that I had been through an important and profound process of healing already. I felt the same way.

27

SAYING THANK YOU

"I'm glad you're here," I told my mom. She'd just arrived from Calgary and was helping me get ready for our thank-you party. I had written an email to Mom and Dad outlining all that was happening on the weekend and they immediately phoned asking if the note was an invitation. My mom had been able to book a flight.

"You know I don't like to miss anything," she said.

"The party will be fun. I've been thinking about it since the day I got home from the hospital."

"Well, I want to thank everyone who helped you just as much as you do," she said.

Because of the exertion of the acupuncture and the physical and emotional preparation for Friday's party, I was in a contemplative space for most of the weekend. Mom said she was surprised at how much calmer I seemed. I was actually sitting and talking with her without getting up to do something, as I would have in the past. Part of my slower nature could be attributed to the fatigue caused by the two previous days, but another part was a change in my approach to activities. I was slower. I felt I could still accomplish what needed to be done, but didn't move frenetically in the way I previously had. Meditation had slowed me down, and so had my understanding that there was no need to rush. I didn't have anywhere to go besides where I was at any given moment. I drove slower, I spoke slower, and I didn't jump into the middle of conversations to add my opinions. Sometimes I worried that my brain wasn't as capable as it once had been of keeping up with the flow of a discussion, but I thought I was just seeing life at a different pace. And I liked it.

I had worried about the party a great deal, though. We had invited almost 60 people and I was still fretting over not having invited some others I'd have liked to. We tried to keep it to those who had helped at the race, family, and friends who had gone out of their way to help. I would have liked to invite more friends who had supported us emotionally and at least some of the nurses from the hospitals as well. As it was, almost everyone came. I had invited Doctors Ofiesh, Morgan, and Fairhurst at the last minute, thinking they probably wouldn't want to be involved in a social event with patients. Dr. Ofiesh was in Toronto and sent his regrets at not being able to attend, but the other two came and had a wonderful time, fitting right in with all the other guests. Dennis Morgan told us that he had never been invited to a party like this and felt honoured to be there. He told Debbie that he was usually able to disassociate himself from his patients since they were either older or unfit, but he was really moved by my situation since we were close in age and in similar family circumstances with children of almost the same ages. Nick Fairhurst seemed to have such a good time that he was almost bubbly in his enthusiasm. When he'd called to accept the invitation, he said that he would be able to stay only half an hour since he and his wife had another function to attend, but they stayed for almost two hours.

> *How do you thank someone*
> *who has taken you from death to life?*

For weeks, I had imagined what I would say at the party. During my meditations the week before, I ran through a speech several times, where I thanked everyone in turn. So that's what I did. I wasn't able to say everything that I had planned to say, but I managed to thank everyone I had wanted to without breaking down entirely. And there were enough laughs to keep the audience from becoming too emotional. I was exhausted after it, but felt as though I had accomplished something that had worried me since I first became cognizant of what had happened. I wanted so much to publicly thank everyone and to throw a party of celebration at the same time. That's what happened. It was a great party.

The following day, an article about my heart attack was published in Victoria's *Times Colonist* newspaper. The writer wanted to tie the story into the Garden City 10K race that Sunday and focus on the Periodical Writers Association of Canada (PWAC), a professional writers' organization I belong to. Many of my friends and colleagues in the group had decided to raise funds for the Heart and Stroke Foundation, the charity for the race, and to participate in the run together in my name. Contrary to what I had told the reporter, the article, title, and page one lead-in all mentioned that I would be walking in the race. I had thought I would start with the PWAC group to show my support, but didn't think I could walk the whole thing. I was a little worried about it, but decided I should at least register for the race, so did that on Saturday.

As it turned out, the day was beautiful and the weather fabulous. Importantly, I managed to actually finish the walk, which was a tremendous lift. I didn't feel tired at all. Lucas ran the race, but the rest of us walked slowly, chatting with each other: Mom, Debbie, Luanne, Raechel, and Leo in the baby jogger. Along the route, several others joined in to offer congratulations and walk with us from time to time.

The ending was incredible. The writers' group was at the finish line cheering us in along with several friends, the newspaper editor who had arranged the story, and another runner who'd had a similar collapse at the end of a race. And suddenly, it seemed, Rachel Staples, Cheryl Wood, Ron Youngash, and John Catterall were right there around us – just as they had been at the end of the race when I'd collapsed. It was a thrilling emotional experience to see them all and to be able to share with them again. They had all been very moved by the party on Friday and seemed to want to be with me as much as I wanted to be with them. It was an unbelievable fitting end to the race.

The weekend truly marked a turning point. I was exhausted on Saturday having gone through the emotions of thanking everyone on Friday. But I felt, at the same time, a sense of closure. Thanking everyone had finalized an accomplishment I had been working towards for weeks. Then completing the race on Sunday added another dimension. Physically I felt wonderful. The exercise did me good, but so did the emotional high of the experience. Even though I didn't run, I completed something that had killed me, as Dr. Greenwood described it. In a way, I was getting back on the horse. But I was doing it differently. All through the race, I marveled at the view, at the smiles on the walkers' faces, at the musicians entertaining along the route, at the absolute perfection of the day. If I'd run, I'd have missed all of that. I realized that I want to run again, but not at the expense of missing what I had noticed for the first time that Sunday. I did feel uncomfortable walking at times. I wanted to run. I wanted to show that I was capable of going faster. But, in the end, it didn't matter.

As we were entering Beacon Hill Park, a former student ran up to me from behind to congratulate me. I couldn't even remember her name, but she told me about her father having bypass surgery a year earlier and about how moved she was to see me out there walking. I realized then, that my walking wasn't just for me. The fact that I was doing it meant something to a number of people. That was a very humbling realization – that I could have some influence, that I could be a symbol. I realized how important it was for me to be walking that day. And I felt elated.

As Paul Taylor, our minister friend, was leaving the party on Friday, he said that, while I was talking, he realized I was expressing and embodying the death and resurrection myth of Christianity. Christ died, was resurrected, and by the message of those events, was able to spread Christianity through the acts of his apostles subsequent to that. The apostles were the community that spread the word. I had talked about community when I was thanking everyone – about the community of support that saved me. Because that community was there, the story of my survival would be told. And there was a message in that story. It wasn't that I thought of myself as Christ-like, but that, as Paul said, the community had a story to spread. This felt important to me: that the story I was living should continue to be told.

28

SUMMER SOLSTICE

"Where are you going?" asked Debbie as I tried to ease out of bed without waking her.

"For a short bike ride," I said.

"Why so early?"

"I'm going to watch the sunrise."

"You are?"

"Don't sound so surprised."

"It's still dark. Be careful."

I'd awakened earlier than usual that morning. It was June 21st, the Summer Solstice. Some friends of mine were holding a Sun Greeting Ceremony at a beach a few miles out of town, but I didn't want to get in the car and drive for half an hour to join them. I decided to ride my bike to another beach, only a 5-minute cycle from our house.

It was 5:00 am and the city was slowly waking. I love riding at night and in the early morning. The streets are deserted and you don't have to be constantly on the lookout for cars driving

too closely. I arrived at the ocean just as the sky was starting to
lighten. The eastern horizon was streaked with light clouds, but I
could already see a pink glow developing through them. I leaned
my bike against a retaining wall, and walked to the water's edge. I
jumped onto a rock that jutted out of the water and squatted into
a seated position without actually sitting on the damp rock. This
felt comfortable. I remembered my uncle telling me once that he
marveled at how, as a child, I could sit in this squatting position
for hours. I rarely squatted now.

> *Why do we forget to take the time*
> *to watch the sun rise?*

I rarely watched sunrises now, either. The glow on the horizon
was slowly brightening. I estimated it would be at least ten minutes before I would actually be able to see the sun itself. I closed
my eyes and listened. Waves gently lapped against the rock in
front of me. What sounded like a pair of geese flew close over-
head, their wings creating a rhythmic swoosh as they passed by
me. Gulls cried nearby. Crows called excitedly. I heard the drone
of a floatplane further out in the strait. I breathed in the sounds
with the fresh sea air and smiled.

When I opened my eyes, the horizon's glow had deepened.
Pink permeated the clouds. Even the snow capping the moun-
tains across the strait to the south held a pinkish hue. I tried to
remember other times I'd sat watching a sunrise like this: once in
the south of France after a double date, days before my reluctant
return to Canada, that became a night of walking and talking

ending up on the Marseilles shoreline facing the east; another at the end of a student exchange to the Maritimes, a group of teenagers willing ourselves to stay awake until the sun burst upon us. Why could I not think of any times more recently? Had I really not watched a sunrise in over 20 years?

The sun didn't burst upon me this time. It slowly emerged through the clouds, the air feeling immediately warmer it seemed. The light reflecting off the ocean increased its intensity. I wanted to stare longer, but knew I couldn't. I wanted to take a photograph, but knew I would never be able to capture this moment through a camera lens. I closed my eyes again and simply tried to remember.

The sound of running footsteps on the gravel beach startled me. I opened my eyes and turned to see a young woman running behind and past me. Slightly embarrassed to be poised so prominently on the rock, I tried to stand, but my legs had stiffened. I couldn't squat like this the way I had been able to when I was young. I watched the woman run along the shore, so intent on her pace that she didn't seem to have noticed me. She looked down at the beach in front of her without glancing out towards the water, oblivious to the sunrise. I'd run along this beach many times in the past, probably unaware of the sunrise as well. For a moment, I thought I should be running too. Instead, I stood up, shook the stiffness from my legs, looked once more across the ocean to the risen sun, and turned toward my bike.

29

ALMOST THERE

"So how are you feeling?" an acquaintance I hadn't seen since before the cardiac arrest asked me one day. "Are you back to normal?"

I was reluctant to respond, "Yes, 100%." Instead I said, "Almost there." The question of whether or not I was back to normal became almost a standard query from people I met. And that became my pat response to the inevitable question.

"Almost there."

As the months passed after my heart attack, my life became busier. In the midst of summer, I was immersed in the activities of life once more. We were spending more time at our cabin, doing more constructing and deconstructing than playing. I longed to do more of the latter. There was a drive in both Debbie and me that led us away, too often, from what was truly important.

But spending more time at the lake, I began to feel stronger. Most of the days were spent building walls, pulling wire through studs, cutting down trees and clearing brush. But I did swim everyday. And one day Lucas and I ventured out on a 45-minute mountain bike ride that got my heart beating as fast as it had in months. I felt good. I felt weary of the responsibilities of the cabin, but I felt comfortable pushing myself physically.

Throughout our time at the lake, though, I worried about my mother. Five months after my cardiac arrest, she called to tell me that she had found a lump on her breast and a biopsy had revealed breast cancer. As she spoke those words, my first impulse was to swallow my emotions and respond with support and positive words of encouragement. But I couldn't. I started to speak, but could only gasp. I started to cry.

At the end of the line from Calgary, my mother's voice dripped concern for me. "Greg? Are you okay? Oh, I'm sorry. I shouldn't have called."

"No," I said fighting to gain control of my emotions. "Of course you should have called. I'm sorry for reacting this way." My heart filled with concern for my mom and anger at this disease that she should never have contracted.

It took me several moments to be able to speak with any clarity. The whole time, my mother kept trying to comfort me, when I should have been comforting her. Finally, I was able to find out that she would be undergoing surgery soon. Her doctor wouldn't know the extent of the surgery needed until they were actually in the operating room, though.

Half way through the summer, we received some good news from her. Without performing a radical mastectomy, the surgeon was able to remove all of the cancerous growth. They found no evidence of the disease in the seven lymph nodes they removed, and she felt strong and confident.

Her diagnosis made me think about the power of disease in our lives. Unexpected ailments can turn our lives around dramatically. I felt as close to pre-January 11th normality as I ever had, but I knew I'd never be the same. Sometimes during our days at the lake, I would become aware of the fact that I hadn't thought about my heart for over an hour. But those times were rare. Finding a rat in our food bin set my heart racing as much as it had on our mountain bike foray. And I feared the stress of facing a rodent and a cabin that required months of work to keep those rodents out was too much for my heart.

How can we gain power over illness?

Until my cardiac arrest, I hadn't realized how truly powerless we can feel in the face of illness. I didn't know if damage to my heart had permanently compromised its operation. I couldn't tell if my arteries were clogging again with plaque. I had no idea what role little stresses in my life played with my overall health. With a broken arm or even a cut finger, we can watch the injury heal. We can't see the bone mend, but we can feel it healing. We can't see our skin repair, but we can, over time, notice the gradual recession of the reddened abrasion. Internally, it's different. The scar on my chest was less prominent, but I didn't know what the occasional flutter of my heart really meant.

And I was still curious about my brain. We played *Trivial*

Pursuit a couple of evenings at the cabin. I'd always prided myself in my ability to recall the useless facts that make up that game. So, I wondered how I would do. Once in awhile, I'd feel frustratingly impaired when I couldn't quickly recall a fact I thought I should know. But at other times, names and events shot through to me from some past knowledge base I couldn't readily identify. Most of these abilities seemed either intact or reconnected. Those reconnections, the vast chasms in my brain that I'd somehow been able to leap, humbled me.

It had taken me time to reach this point. For months, I'd felt deeply worried about my brain capacity, even my ability to make simple decisions. I would stare at all of the boxes of crackers in a grocery store aisle unable to decide which brand to choose. I found it difficult to transfer a number someone told me over the phone to a piece of paper. I couldn't concentrate on a subject for any length of time when listening to someone. I'd feel exhausted after what would usually be a normal day's activities. The automated voice at the other end of the phone line would keep repeating, "I'm sorry, you have not entered a valid response," as I tried to pay bills over the phone but couldn't remember, let alone input fast enough, the required numbers for the machine.

A book I read listed some of the effects of even a mild head injury: fatigue, forgetfulness, difficulty doing more than one thing at a time, and inability to make decisions or concentrate. I'd experienced all of these nagging frustrations but was subtly ignoring them, not wanting to dwell on them. Were they simply signs of aging? Or was my brain permanently impaired?

The book talked about students who had been above average

in their school achievements before suffering a brain injury, but were suddenly mired in average accomplishments after a head trauma. They felt frustrated at having to work much harder at something that previously had been very easy. That's the way I felt. More and more of what I tried to do felt like a chore. I had to work at remembering appointments, I strained to recall examples off the top of my head while conversing, and I struggled to find even the most obvious synonym when trying to add variety to my writing.

I had to acknowledge that what I was going through was real. I had suffered a brain injury – an event that was completely separate from my cardiac arrest and surgery. I had to let myself accept that fact and try to deal with it by relearning what I had lost. Even though I was responding "Almost there" when asked if I was back to normal, I needed to realize that I'd never be completely "there." I had a new normal now.

Many experts believe that there is no such thing as a "minor" head injury. Any injury to the brain is major. The portion of a brain damaged by injury never recovers. Somehow though, and scientists don't know exactly how this happens, the brain finds new portions of itself to compensate for the damaged parts. I'd literally felt that happening. My brain function would always be impaired, though. A scar on my chest proved that I had gone through heart surgery, but I had no physical evidence to show that there was ever damage to my brain. Being without adequate oxygen for 20 minutes, my brain must have suffered. Its repair had been remarkable but I had to admit there was damage inflicted.

All my life, I'd been defined by my intelligence. In elementary school, classmates would try to copy my work. In junior high school, my peers referred to me as the one who read, the one who got A's, the nerd. In high school, my marks allowed me to be the graduating class valedictorian. In university, I won a fellowship to do graduate work. Even when I was in my first year of teaching, a student told one of my colleagues that he'd like to be as athletic as another of our colleagues and as smart as Mr. Marchand. I was the brain, not the brawn.

Now my brain had been damaged. The reality of that affected me. But I tried to fight it. The way Terry Fox fought his cancer. The way Stephen Hawking fights his ALS. The way Muhammad Ali fights his Parkinson's disease. My battle was small compared to theirs, but my biggest battle was the one to survive, and I'd accomplished that. Now I had to battle the lack of self-confidence and drive I seemed to have at times. I had to battle the frustrations of not being able to do everything I wanted to do. I had to battle the pressure I felt to succeed and accomplish. I had to battle the portion of my brain that tried to shut down when I most needed it, that vacillated in the middle of decisions, that struggled to recall.

30

RATTLING MY CAGE

"They're tiring now, keep up the pressure," called out the coach from the opposing team. "You've got them where you want them."

In September, seven months after my bypass surgery, I had taken on more teaching responsibilities and had volunteered to coach Raechel's school soccer team. I had been coaching her community league team, but had to stop after my cardiac arrest. The girls had been doing well, had lost only one game and had earned a spot in the playoffs. In our first match, we played a team fairly comparable to ours in skill level, but who were very aggressive. Their team was being charged with fouls frequently for shoulder checking, elbowing, and aggressive tackling. Even Raechel was knocked to the ground once by a hard tackle.

The team's coach was just as aggressive as his players. He prowled the sidelines, crossing in front of our bench several times, calling to his team continuously. He wasn't simply coaching and offering encouragement, but shouting out comments that disparaged our team. All of my team's parents were dumbfounded by his blatant put-downs.

At half time, I walked up to him, shook his hand, deliberately didn't let go of his hand so that I could look directly into his eyes, and calmly asked if he could keep his comments directed to his own team without making reference to ours.

He laughed and said, "I'm just coaching."

Shortly after the second half began, one of his players knocked one of ours over so forcefully that she had the wind knocked out of her. Poor Katie was in tears trying to breathe as she lay on the field. We were awarded a direct shot because the referee deemed the infraction deliberate.

After I attended to Katie and substituted another player on, I went over to the coach and said much more forcefully than I had the first time I'd spoken to him, "Your girls wouldn't be so aggressive if you were less aggressive on the sidelines."

He smiled and said, "They're just having fun."

When is outrage healthy?

I was furious, and surprised at my fury. Since my cardiac arrest, I'd been very low-key emotionally. In some ways, I'd deliberately tried to maintain a calm disposition and at the same time, felt that my demeanour was simply part of the changes I'd gone through. I didn't feel as aggressive as I once had, and I didn't want to be.

At times over the preceding few months, I wondered if I'd become too passive. I feared that I wouldn't have the wherewithal to even protect my family in the event of some sort of emergency. My passivity had made me feel somewhat helpless.

That's why I was surprised at my reaction to this coach. I felt the need to protect the girls on my soccer team and I didn't back down. In fact he did. After my second comment to him, he stopped his sideline tirades almost completely. Our team seemed to gather momentum from the incident. We were down 1–0 at the time and did everything but score the tying goal, keeping the ball in their end for most of the second half. I was overcome with pride at their efforts.

That morning, I had read my horoscope in the newspaper. I rarely read it – almost never do – but this one interested me. It said, "Librans are like big cats you see at the zoo; they look nice and cuddly but if you rattle their cage you could find yourself minus an arm. Someone, somewhere is about to discover what a dangerous creature you can be when roused. After that they should keep their distance."

After I read the horoscope, I thought, "This doesn't apply to me. I'm much too calm these days to be 'roused.'" I thought of the horoscope, though, right after the game. On the one hand, I felt good that I was still capable of protecting. I felt like my old self in a way that I hadn't for months. At the same time, I wondered how healthy it was for me to be roused in that way. I still had no idea what caused the blockages in my arteries. I may have a predisposition to stress that can result in the constricted passages I developed around my heart. Coaching soccer may not have been in my best interest.

That was my biggest frustration – not knowing. Not knowing

what caused the blockages. Not knowing whether they could become blocked again. Not knowing what to do to keep them clear.

Our health is so fragile and elusive. We really don't know what's going on inside our bodies and we don't truly know whether what we do to our bodies is good or not. Sometimes I felt like a remote operator of a being completely removed from me. When our car had broken down recently and even the mechanics couldn't figure out what was wrong, I was reminded of myself. The mechanics replaced a few computer chips hoping they'd solve the operating problems of my car. Surgeons replaced a few arteries in my chest hoping they'd solve the operating problems of my heart.

31

TRYING TO REGAIN
CONFIDENCE

"I don't understand this," a student said to me.

"You don't understand what?" I asked.

"Why I have to write Kim and me. I've always been told I should say Kim and I."

"Well, that all depends on whether you need to use the subjective or objective case of the pronoun in that part of the sentence."

"I still don't understand."

"Let me try to explain."

September had come, and I had begun to teach more. Often the teaching was more challenging than I was expecting. I sometimes found it difficult to explain concepts that I once understood entirely. And periodically, in the midst of my teaching and seemingly from out of nowhere, I'd be unexpectedly struck with the profound realization that I'd actually had open-heart surgery. Of course, I thought about it all the time. But once in a while, the reality of my health-affected life gave me pause. It had seemed so matter-of-fact to me while I was in the hospital. I completely trusted my doctors and family, believing that I needed to go through the procedure that I was about to experience. I didn't remember feeling any fear at all as I waited for the operation. I was swept along in a wave of procedures that I really had no control over.

I wasn't really sure that I completely understood what I'd gone through. At times I wanted simply to carry on as before. I read about men going back to work mere weeks after their bypasses and marveled at their resiliency. At the same time, I wondered whether they'd given themselves the opportunity to contemplate their close encounters with death.

I felt caught in that dichotomy. I'd begun to teach again. I was coaching Raechel's soccer team. I was organizing grad meetings for her class. I was trying to keep the household functioning. And I was following my dream of writing.

In the midst of all that, however, I wondered whether I'd come to grips with this whole experience. Talking to my friend Mick on the phone from Calgary one night, I wondered whether I was skirting too many issues. He questioned whether I was cognizant of the enormity of what I'd gone through. I'd been wondering that too.

I wondered about the functioning of my brain as well. Simple analysis exhausted me. Extended conversations left me daydreaming. My powers of concentration and ability to reason didn't feel as sharp as they used to. So I wondered if writing about anything was almost futile.

My self-confidence had crumbled. I knew the way I presented myself in the classroom was different than it used to be and I knew the erosion of my self-esteem was a large part of that change. I used to feel completely on top of the subject area I was presenting. Now I feared that uncertainty came across to the students.

I could feel those erosions, but did they exist in reality? The more I felt I'd lost confidence, the less confident I felt. I was afraid of creating a self-fulfilling prophesy – that I was less able simply because I kept thinking I was.

What do we do when we can't find the answer?

One day, I was asked to explain a grammar concept in my adult education class. The student who asked the question was a woman about my age who'd recently moved to Canada from Asia and was upgrading her English skills. Her strength as a student was only matched by her enthusiasm. Her questions were always thoughtful and often beyond the ken of many of the other students. The answer to this particular question didn't come readily to me. As I'd learned to do when confronted by questions or problems that I couldn't respond to immediately, I started to talk about the question, allowing my brain to catch up to the answer as it formulated in my head. It would feel as though I was coaxing the answer out of my consciousness. I knew the answer was somewhere in my brain. I just had to give it time to come to the surface. This process would usually work. It would take time, but I generally succeeded. I never admitted this slight failing to anyone. Someone who knew me well might observe my groping for an answer, but I'd learned to hide the clambering around talk. Sometimes it was an exhausting process, but usually it was successful.

So I started responding to this student's question in that roundabout fashion. This time, though, the answer didn't come. The more I talked around the question, the further away from the correct response I moved. I was embarrassed. I began to perspire. But I kept trying. By the time I finished my rambling, I knew I had not only failed to answer the question, but I had probably confused the entire class in the process. The student was gracious. She nodded politely, but I knew I hadn't helped. And I felt as though I had betrayed her confidence in me as a teacher.

That evening, I fretted over my response. When I checked out the concept in a grammar text at home, I discovered that my rambling was not just inaccurate but incorrect. The next day, I began the class by apologizing. I told the students about my cardiac arrest, my brain injury, and my difficulties in being able to come up with quick answers at times. I assured them that they weren't getting a shoddy education. The answers were there. They just might take a little longer than normal to come to the surface for me. The class couldn't have been more supportive. They were intrigued by my story and were more than willing to help me in helping them to learn. These students were themselves a blessing.

The recovery of my brain was so much different than the recovery of my body. As I felt stronger, I knew my body was healing.

As I ran more, I had physical proof that I was strengthening. But how could I gauge my brain's recovery? Nobody knew what was going on inside my head. I couldn't turn to a doctor and ask, "How much brain capacity did I lose? When will it all return?"

I felt stymied by all this. I wondered how healthy it was for me to even speculate too much about the whole event and my recovery. I worried about being worried. But my chest still hurt, my heart still palpitated, and my brain was still too fuzzy. I wondered what was going on in my body every minute of the day.

32

WHAT ALMOST DYING TAUGHT ME

"So what did you learn this year?'
My friend's sudden question caught me by surprise.
"What do you mean?" I asked.

"You almost died a year ago," he said. "You must have learned something this year thinking about the event."

I had most certainly thought about the event. In fact, I had thought of little else during the year. But I hadn't contemplated the lessons of almost dying. So I sat down. I thought. And I wrote.

I learned that life is tenuous. I learned that we can't count on anything staying the same. I learned that lack of health can stymie ambition, creativity, and achievement.

I learned that family is paramount, that prayer has power, that simplicity beats complexity, and that people waste time in pursuits that are often meaningless. I learned that we can see much more by walking than by running, that we need very little to survive comfortably, and that it's easier to be kind than cruel. I learned that people respond positively to goodness and that everyone is searching for something.

I learned that there are several paths to understanding. I learned that the flight of a bird is as moving as the smile of a child and that many people work too hard. I learned to sleep more.

I learned to play more. I learned that time missed being with your children is time lost and that friendship transcends time and distance. I learned that concerns about health are universal and that the endorphin rush from exercise can be as powerful and as dangerous as morphine. I learned that we don't really know what's going on inside our bodies. I learned that doctors don't really know what's going on inside our bodies. I learned that stress is as debilitating as disease.

I learned that the brain can heal over time, that sunshine both heals and harms, and that the heart is more than a muscle.

I learned that there is as much art in medicine as there is science. I learned that many of our most profound setbacks are completely unexpected. I learned that change teaches us, that failure teaches us, that time spent reflecting is time well spent, and that the contemplation gained from raking leaves can't be duplicated by a leaf blower. I learned that wearing my heart on my sleeve is better than keeping emotions in check. I learned to cry.

I learned to smile. I learned to listen. I learned to sit. I learned that time is precious and that television robs us of time. I learned that writing can heal and that children give us hope. I learned that time passes too quickly as we age. I learned that the true pleasures of life don't come in megabytes or horsepower and that the closer we come to death, the clearer life becomes.

I learned that the truest messages come from the unlikeliest sources and that feeling loved is more powerful than death. I learned that death isn't negative. I learned that our fear of death is really fear of an unlived life.

I learned that as we move away from death, we miss the messages of life: that life is not easy when we're too immersed in it, but life is simple when we treat it simply.

33

ONE YEAR LATER

The day had arrived: one year after I died and was brought back to life. I felt celebratory. The renewed life I'd been given beat within me through my bypassed heart. I felt more alive than I had in months. The weekend helped that to happen. It was a turning point, a hurdle to overcome, a pinnacle. The annual Harriers 8K race at the Saanichton Fairgrounds was taking place that weekend, and I knew I had to run it again.

My sister Colette and her family flew out from Calgary on Friday to be with us for the weekend. Their arrival began what was truly a celebration. I had worried about their coming when I first learned about it the week before. I felt tired of life focusing on me so much. I wanted the focus to shift. I felt like everyone else in my family deserved to have some of the attention I'd been receiving for so long. But the weekend was one of those times when events coalesced to help move my healing forward.

On the morning of January 11th, my family greeted me with our traditional birthday ritual: breakfast in bed. They had decided that this was my second birthday, the day of my rebirth into a new life, and they wanted to celebrate. They even had a present for me. Debbie later told me that the whole idea for a morning birthday party came from the kids. They wheeled in a huge present for me: a rolling desk chair that offered me luxurious comfort as I wrote.

They understood my need to be writing. They'd all seen me write all their lives. Lucas once told me about a memory he has of my writing. When I was writing my MA thesis, I would often work late into the night in his room since there was no other space in the house with a desk. The usual pattern was for me to read to him in our bed as a bedtime ritual then tuck him into bed in our room so that I could use his room to work. After an evening of writing, I'd carry him, soundly sleeping, back to his own bed before I went to sleep. One night, though, he snuck back to his room and climbed into his bed hiding under the covers so that I didn't see him. He says that at one point I even sat on the edge of his bed to read something I'd written, oblivious to the fact that he was there in the room with me.

Raechel had always written as well. She'd already filled several journals full of her musings. She kept lists of things to accomplish almost from the day she had learned to write. On the card that accompanied my present, she'd written about the race, imagining my thoughts and feelings. Part of it read,

> *Excruciating moments for some*
> *Exist as a light beyond your reach*
> *To guide you to find further truths*
> *Beyond the heart, the life, the eye.*

Raechel's writing always plumbed the depth of her own compassion in a way that had become a lesson to me and a model for my own writing.

Luanne had been planning what she called a "life party" for me on Saturday evening as well. I was looking forward to it, but I feared too much attention there also. From my 40th birthday party at her house 15 months earlier until the thank-you party for those who helped at the race, much of her energy – like Debbie's and the rest of my family's – had been centred on me. I didn't want that. But the party was a profound experience. It was thankfully low key, and highlighted by my friend Don and brother-in-law Keith reprising two songs: Keith's birthday song for me that he'd written for my 40th and Don's song "I Believe" that he'd written last January and performed at our thank-you party. The opening verses to the song tell the story of my collapse:

> *There's a story, and it fell at the finish line,*
> *On a cold and broken winter's day.*
> *I can hardly believe the story is mine.*
> *But it was carried by a thousand faithful hands.*
> *They gave it back to me.*
> *That's what I believe.*
> *It's what you believe that keeps you strong.*
> *It's what you believe that helps you hang on.*

He added an extra verse using lines from a column I'd written about what I'd learned in this past year. It was beautiful. The meal was great – all low-fat food – and the opportunity to celebrate with those I love was uplifting.

Can you ever go back?

Sunday was the race. I had worried about the weather. I knew I couldn't run if it was close to being as cold as it had been the year before. We awoke to a balmy 6°C with a drizzly rain and we all drove out to the Saanichton Fairgrounds. It was the first time I'd been there since the year before.

I tried to recall the road leading up to the fairgrounds as we turned off Stelly's Cross Road. I had written that the road was gravel and remembered a gravely image from my acupuncture treatment. It does have exposed gravel on its surface, tarred in place. I had remembered a finish line sign in my vision and there it was, hanging across the gravel entrance as we drove up to the parking lot. Nothing else struck me as reminiscent. In fact, the day was very much a celebration of life and not a reliving of a collapse and near death as I had feared it might be.

We found Cheryl Wood, the CPR-performing anesthetist, soon after we entered the crowded hall. She was bouncing around, her multi-coloured socks pulled up to her knees and a pair of bells tied to her laces. Every time she moved, she rang. John Catterall, who'd led the prayers over me the year before, arrived shortly before we set out. His speed could have kept him near the front of the pack, but he wanted to run with us as well. And, of course, Lucas was there, pleased to be part of the group.

Outside the hall, the members of my men's group greeted me. My friend Dan MacIsaac appeared with his friend, Dr. Dan O'Connell. They had both been at the race the year before. Dr. Dan started to tell me about how dead he had thought I looked the previous year as I lay on the roadside, but surprisingly, I didn't want to hear that. I felt too buoyed by the energy of the day.

We found a spot near the back of the pack, and just before the start, Rob Reid arrived pulling his young sons along. He ran into the fairgrounds building to drop the boys off at the child-minding centre and got back to us just before the start. He managed to pull off his warm-up pants just as the race began.

I felt a little cold at first. The rain chilled my arms and hands making me wish I had worn a long-sleeved shirt and gloves. But soon it didn't matter. I was warm and thrilled. As we ran, I marveled at the comfort of running this race. We took the first half very slowly, chatting the whole time and trying to explain to everyone around us why Rob, the nationally-ranked marathoner, was so far back in the pack. I let Cheryl set the pace at first, but soon Lucas and I were moving ahead a bit. We were running at a slower pace than we usually run, and I felt like letting it out. At the same time, I didn't want to lose anyone and realized there was no need to run any faster. I had nothing to prove. We passed a flooded field by the side of the road and a vague image of skaters slipped through my mind. Then someone mentioned seeing people skating on the same field the year before.

When we looped past the road leading up to the fairgrounds, the crowd lining the road was wonderful. Debbie, Raechel and Leo were at the bottom of the hill, Debbie snapping photos and calling out, "I didn't think you'd be here so soon." My sisters and their families were further down the road. At the turn before an uphill climb, all the guys from the men's group were poised to cheer us on.

The rest of the race was pure fun. I didn't once feel tired. We slowed often to let Cheryl catch up with us after she had stopped to tie her shoe and have a drink. But the last half was exhilarating.

Turning down the road leading to the final turn, I had a moment of anxiety realizing that the last kilometre was longer that it appeared at first. But the crowd and the anticipation of finishing spurred me on. I had feared the final uphill push toward the finish line. Michael Greenwood's acupuncture treatments had made me realize that the year before I had pushed that final sprint too hard. When Lucas and I ran in the previous months, we had always walked up the final hill towards home. I hadn't wanted to push. But the hill at the end of the race was easy. There was no one to try to pass at the end. I felt no desire to try pushing myself harder.

Rob ran ahead of us wanting to relive the year before when he high-fived me just before the finish line. He did it again. Cheryl and I were side-by-side as we crossed the line. I reached over and grasped her hand as we crossed at exactly the same moment.

In anticipating the finish line of this race over the previous few weeks, I'd imagined myself bursting into tears at the end. But I felt no sense of sadness at all. My only emotion was ecstasy. I was blissfully happy.

I stood in the rain hugging everyone as Debbie and a *Times Colonist* photographer snapped photos. I wasn't tired. I didn't want to get out of the rain. I felt only a profound joy and an enormous thrill in being able to share this moment with so many people.

The thrill continued into the hall. I had been worried about everyone sticking around for so long to endure the extended awards distribution. But my family and friends stayed. Before the awards began, the announcer called Rob up to the stage. Rob began by talking about the heart and led into a description of last year's race and my collapse at the end. He then called me up to receive a special award. I walked up to the stage to an incredible ovation. I'd never felt anything like it. Over 600 people applauded in a sustained expression of their joy. I was stunned.

Rob then introduced the award as a trophy in my name to be presented each year to a cardiac patient who uses the race as part of his or her rehabilitation. He then turned the microphone over to me. Holding back tears, I thanked him, the Prairie Inn Harriers Running Club for the award, and the support of the running community. I was completely overwhelmed by the presentation. It was a stunning conclusion to an amazing day.

What does it take to live life to the fullest?

When we arrived home, I went downstairs and, for some reason, checked the messages on my office phone line. I rarely do that on weekends. There was a message from a reporter at the *Times Colonist* newspaper asking to phone her right away. The photographer had returned with his photos and she wanted to write about the event and my story. I told her the details.

On the front page of the paper the next morning, readers were greeted with a picture of Cheryl and me running and grinning as I reached out to give Rob a high-five, as well as a story about my running the race a year after my cardiac arrest.

It was an important day even though I almost hadn't run the

race. I knew how much Debbie feared my running it, but I also knew how much I wanted and needed to run. The run allowed me to experience another of the enormous leaps I had made during the year – a physical, emotional, and even spiritual leap. I felt healthy, vibrant, and alive. And I had run the race differently, feeling no sense of competition, simply the joy of running. One year after my "death," I knew I was going to live, perhaps for a long time, maybe a short time, but definitely a full time.

BASKING IN THE GLOW

My spring break from teaching school is almost over. It's been a wonderful time for me. I've rested, I've read, and I've written. I wrote the last chapter of my book today. I tried to follow the pattern I'd established when I wrote the bulk of my manuscript, my back against the headboard of my bed, my legs stretched in front of me, and the computer on my lap. The ritual of being in the same position and writing in a pattern that had been successful in the past helped. I finished it. The sense of accomplishment buoys me. I've completed a task that began more than a dozen years ago and has been calling to me for completion ever since.

Our bedroom looks more like a study today. Books crowd my bedside table and old journals of mine spill across the floor. The bed itself is a sea of crumpled sheets and blankets.

I strip the sheets from the bed and take them downstairs to the washing machine. I load them into the washer and walk back upstairs to the bedroom. I try to bring some order to the chaos, return books to the shelf, stack my journals into a corner, and return the pens and pencils tossed on my dresser to the desk in our extra bedroom down the hall.

This has been a productive break for me. Leo had wanted to travel more than we did. He wanted to visit Lucas whose band is playing in Morocco for the next four months, or Raechel whose travels have led her to Thailand. I've talked to them both recently. Lucas is enjoying his time in Morocco with his band and the opportunity to perform every day and earn enough money to save a little each week. And Raechel loves Thailand. Like Leo, I would have enjoyed traveling to visit them during the break as well, but I know I had to complete this. Writing was more than a simple exercise these last few weeks. It was the opportunity to bring peace to my soul, to bring clarity to my mind, and to bring relief to my heart.

The writing process itself has given me some perspective to my year of dying, living, and healing. Because I've been close to dying, I've learned that we have nothing to fear in death. What lies beyond this realm is simply another segment of life's journey. I've felt too connected to those I've known who have passed over to believe that nothing else exists, that life in this world is finite.

Yet there is much in this world to keep me here. I don't feel a temptation to slip any bonds at all. The comfort of life right now sustains me. The joy of my existence often overwhelms me. The glories of this world astound me.

Our world is made up of the cycle of birth and rebirth. Every form of life on this Earth goes through that cycle: "Mighty oaks from tiny acorns grow." At the end of its life, the struggling salmon literally spawns new life as it returns to the spot at which it was hatched and then dies. I once visited Hiroshima and marveled at the flowers and grasses around the shell of a building left standing at the impact point of the atomic bomb, its skeleton a reminder to us that life continues in the face of devastation.

Our lives give rise to that same spirit of sustainability. We are not the end just as the atomic bomb was not the end. Individually, each of our cells contains the necessary DNA to replicate our bodies. Those same cells die and replace themselves every day just as our spirits continue to live in the memories of those who remain here after our passing.

Life is precious and perpetual. It thrives despite our seeming lack of effort to support it at times. The lungs of a smoker become completely normal two years after that smoker stops his habit, the body longing to be healthy again. Our bodies are as bountiful as the planet on which we live. Like the planet, we are constantly moving toward life, not death.

For a year after my cardiac arrest, I worked for recovery. The recovery of my physical body was manifested when I crossed the finish line of the same race one year later, holding the hand of one of the people who had initially saved my life. The recovery of my cognitive abilities became evident to me when I was able to once again teach an English class. The recovery of my spirituality is ongoing. I learned from my year that our lives are a quest to recover the spiritual within us. Contrary to what I remember from the teachings of my Catholic upbringing, I don't believe we are born with original sin. On the contrary, the miracle I've witnessed in the births I've been lucky enough to be part of has convinced me that we are all born into a state of original grace, not sin. We are born spiritual beings in a temporal world. The spiritual part of our lives is just as real as the temporal. And just as our physical bodies move inevitably toward health, our spiritual selves long to return to that grace, to the spiritual beings we truly are.

Struggling to recover my physical norms, I thought I had to abandon the spiritual realities that I'd been presented with when I nearly died. Slowly, I've been allowing all three to coexist: the physical, the cognitive, and the spiritual. I continue to nourish the physical by running. Interestingly, that running is now becoming a link to all three aspects for me. The oxygen that replenishes my brain when I run helps my brain cells to thrive. More and more studies show that exercise is one of the keys to brain health. Exercise helps us live longer and aids memory, cognition, and concentration. And my running is part of my spiritual quest as well. Because I run slower now, I see more. I try to run in the forest and on trails more than on pavement as I used to. I often stop in the midst of a run to listen to the birds, or marvel at the view, or appreciate the freshness of the air. I rarely run races now. I have nothing to prove by running anymore. I would much rather run by myself, with my children, or with a friend than I would with hundreds or even thousands of others.

I did run a race recently, though, with Raechel. Despite my years of racing, I had never run a half marathon. Raechel wanted to try the distance and asked me if I would like to join her. So we did run with thousands of others that day. But, for me, the only two people running that race were my daughter and I. The beauty of the half marathon is that it's not so long that your body begins to feel as though it's shutting down from exertion and lack of hydration, yet it's long enough that to complete the distance feels like an achievement.

Raechel and I felt as though we'd accomplished something that bound us when we finished. It was challenging and exhilarating and an endeavour we will always share. Running for me now is more about sharing than striving, more about living than dying, more about breathing fragrances than gasping for oxygen, more about reaching for heights than pounding pavement, more about communion than competing, more meditating than focusing, more smiles than miles, more ecstasy than anxiety.

When is it safe just to let go?

When the laundry has been washed, I decide to hang it on the line. It's a beautiful day, the sun shining warmly. A slight breeze pushes the sheets into a slow-motion dance as I pin them to the clothesline. They won't take long to dry. It's allergy season, and the pollen in the air will undoubtedly settle on the sheets as they rustle in the wind. I can just feel my allergies begin to erupt in me these days. But Debbie, who's not affected by allergies, loves the smell of laundry fresh from the line. If I sneeze a couple of times in bed it won't matter.

By mid-afternoon the sheets have dried completely. I bring them inside and take them upstairs to remake the bed, being careful to tuck the corners in and straighten the quilt cover until it lies wrinkle free on the bed, the indentation of the spot where I'd sat while writing no longer apparent.

In the evening, Debbie goes to bed before me. She's tired. She's been back to school a week already, not granted the same luxury of an extended spring break that Leo and I have had. I finally climb into bed beside her. She's already asleep and I try to lie still, breathing in the freshness of the laundered sheets. Immediately my eyes start to water and my nose begins to run. I try to stifle a sneeze, not wanting to wake Debbie. I reach for a tissue on my bedside table and grab it just as a sneeze wracks my chest. Debbie stirs beside me. This isn't going to work, I realize.

I slowly slide out of bed and walk down the hall to the spare bedroom, sneezing repeatedly. It used to be Raechel's room but now houses Lucas's old futon bed, a desk, our computer and a printer. Next to the printer is the freshly printed copy of my manuscript, as complete as it can be for now.

I lie down on the futon, pull the blanket over me, and lean against the pillow. It doesn't take long for me to stop sneezing and start breathing freely again. The pollen on the sheets was obviously too much.

The futon rests below a large, eastern-facing window. In the winter, the window rattles in its frame with every gust of wind. It's a cool spring night, but the air drifting through the cracks in the old windowpane is refreshing. I gaze out the window into the darkened sky. Wisps of clouds drift by, and through them I can make out the filtered light of what looks like a full moon. The sky begins to lighten as the clouds covering the moon disperse. This feels lovely. I breathe deeply, the lack of pollen in these bed sheets a comfort to my lungs.

As my body begins to relax, my legs start to shake. Then my torso quivers and lurches upward. Since my last acupuncture treatment, my body responds to relaxation, especially as I'm falling asleep or during meditation, by shaking in the same way as it does during the treatments. Lying next to Debbie at night, I try to control the shaking or at least minimize it. Tonight I let go. My whole body begins to shake. My legs pulsate up and down, my head rolls quickly back and forth as my chest bounces against the bed. Just as Michael Greenwood encourages me during acupuncture, I try to release, to let my body go.

The shaking continues for what seems like minutes then abruptly stops. I lie still, my breath coming in gulps. As my breathing slows, my mind starts to drift. I begin to sense a pulsating blackness around me. The blackness begins to grow as it starts to surround me. I'm reminded of the feeling I had with the night terrors of my youth as an undefined fear begins to settle in my chest. I start to worry as my breathing increases and my heartbeat quickens. But then I stop. Instead of worrying about my heart and fighting the fear, I let it slide over and through me. As I do, the blackness slowly subsides and with it, the fear that had begun to creep in.

With my eyes still closed, I see twirls of green, purple, and amber. White shapes float by and I imagine myself drifting. Suddenly I see myself on the back of a giant bird. It looks like an eagle. Its back is covered in what looks like a patterned sweater or vest. I'm reminded of a picture I have of my grandfather taken when he was about the age I am now. He's smiling at the camera and wearing a thick sweater just like the one I imagine myself clinging to.

The eagle starts to fly and I feel as though I'm flying with it, my arms wrapped around its back and the sweater. We drift above the city, over Vancouver Island, up the coast of the Mainland toward Haida Gwaii and further north. We soar higher and higher until I see the entire west coast of Canada, then North America and beyond. The whole Northern Hemisphere comes into view as we drift higher. Then we stop. I see clouds swirling below us that almost block out my view of the Earth. It's a glorious sight.

As I'm looking down, I become aware of presences around me. I sense who they are more than see them. But they're tangible to me: my grandfather, my grandmother, my uncle, Father Leo. Their individual presences feel strong, completely real to me; and their collective presence feels profound. I smile. And from the whole of my heart, the depth of my soul, I thank them.

I feel a tear drip down my cheek and slowly become conscious of where I am, lying in my son's old bed in my daughter's old room, my younger son in the room next door, my wife down the hall. I open my eyes. Through the tears brimming in both eyes now, I see the moon through a cloudless sky. I marvel at its brightness. I close my eyes again and fall asleep, basking in the glow of the full moon.

ACKNOWLEDGEMENTS

This book has been 14 years in the making, so many friends and family have had a hand in its creation.

For those who read early drafts and offered insightful suggestions including Luanne Marchand, Don Chambers, Terence Young, Patricia Young, Jennifer Fraser, Jay Connelly, Susan Macdonald, Dorothy Hawes, Janice McCachen, Julie Salisbury, Beth Allan, Cynthya Cenciarini, Zia Cole, Greg Marion, Linn McKeown, Harold Rhenish, Rosemary Neering, Rob Reid and Peter Tongue, I am indebted for your encouragement and guidance.

For my doctors who have given me ongoing health support over the years, Nick Fairhurst, Denis Morgan and Michael Greenwood, I am forever grateful.

For the members of my men's group, Don Chambers, Alan Jones, Jim LaMorte, Denton Pendergast, Trevor Smyth and Keith Watson, you keep me sane. Special thanks to Denton for his help on the book's cover design.

For Bruce and Marsha Batchelor at Agio Publishing House, I thank you for creatively guiding me through the publication process.

For my lifesaving angels, Cheryl Wood, Rachel Staples, Ron Youngash, Dan Baker and John Catterall, I owe you everything.

For my parents, Pat and Lou, and my sisters, Luanne, Colette and Allison, you are the foundation of my life.

And for my immediate family, Debbie, Lucas, Raechel and Leo, you are the joy of my heart and the ballast of my soul.

ABOUT THE AUTHOR

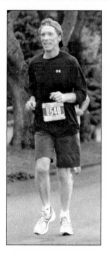

Gregory Marchand has been a runner and competitive athlete all his life. Since suffering a cardiac arrest and subsequently undergoing open-heart surgery in 1998, his running has continued to be a major focus in his life but now as a source of wellness and spiritual growth rather than competition. An educator and counsellor for over 25 years, Marchand is also a prolific freelance writer, having published over 100 magazine and newspaper articles. He and his wife, Debbie, live on Vancouver Island and are newly-hatched empty nesters with three grown children.

Visit Gregory Marchand's website at www.gregorymarchand.com

CPSIA information can be obtained at www.ICGtesting.com
Printed in the USA
LVOW122337280812

296378LV00002B/2/P